DEDICATION

It is with great pleasure and profound gratitude that I dedicate this work to my teachers, colleagues and friends in the Emergency Department of Egleston Children's Hospital in Atlanta. I spent four wonderful years there learning how to take better care of kids. Yet above all I learned to appreciate their love of and devotion to the never-ending stream of children who came through those always open doors. From Department Director to Environmental Services, all were equally dedicated to taking care of these children. The period I was there was a magical time when nurses, residents, paramedics, attendings, respiratory therapists, and fellows all worked together, putting aside disciplinary rivalries to contribute from their strengths, learn from their weaknesses, and make that place a better one for children through the synergy of their talents and experiences.

Guy H. Haskell

For Jeremiah, Katie, and Sarah

Marianne Gausche-Hill

EDITORS

Guy H. Haskell, Ph.D., NREMT-P
Director, Emergency Medical and Safety Services Consultants, Bloomington, Indiana
Paramedic, Bedford Regional Medical Center, Bedford, Indiana

Marianne Gausche-Hill, MD, FACEP
Professor, Department of Medicine, David Geffen School of Medicine, UCLA
Professor, Emergency Medicine, Director of EMS and the EMS and Pediatric Emergency
Medicine Fellowships, Harbor-UCLA Medical Center

ASSOCIATE EDITOR

Mariann M. Manno, M.D., FAAP
Associate Professor of Pediatrics, Director of the Division of Pediatric Emergency Medicine,
University of Massachusetts Medical School

CONTRIBUTING AUTHORS

Cheryl A. Coyle, RN, BSN, CCRN, CFRN, CEN, EMT
Life Flight Medical Crew Chief
University of Massachusetts Memorial Health Care

Cheryl A. Haskell, M.A.
Assistant Director
Marine Educational Services
Bloomington, Indiana

Captain Robert C. Krause, EMT-P
Toledo Fire and Rescue

Robert L. Palmer, PA-C, NREMT-P
Boston Medflight

William T. Zempsky, M.D.
Associate Director, Assistant Professor, Department of Pediatrics, Division of Pediatric
Emergency Medicine, University of Connecticut and Connecticut Children's Medical Center

Property Laws of a Toddler

~ Anonymous ~

If I like it, it's mine

If it's in my hand, it's mine

If I had it a little while ago, it's mine

If it's mine, it must not ever appear to be yours in any way

If I'm doing or building something, all the pieces are mine

If I saw it first, it's mine

If it looks just like mine, it's mine

If you're playing with something and you put it down, it automatically becomes mine

If it's broken, it's yours

INTRODUCTION

Pediatric advanced life support has become such an integral part of emergency care in the United States it is hard to believe that it has been only seventeen years since the first PALS course was offered in the fall of 1988. The abundance of textbooks and courses in pediatric resuscitation currently being produced belie the paucity of concern and resources available for the care of critically ill children at the time that first course was offered. We can recall the spate of newspaper articles decrying the care our children were receiving, the lack of pediatric equipment in our rescue squads and emergency departments, and the inadequate training of our personnel, from first responder to physician, in dealing with pediatric emergencies.

There was a remarkable response to these reports, both at the national and the local levels. Funding was provided by the federal government to establish Emergency Medical Services for Children (EMS-C), a program that has now touched every state in the Union. Research projects were planned, needs were assessed, equipment was purchased, child safety programs were initiated, and courses were developed.

Among the most successful programs created during this period was the American Heart Association's (AHA) Pediatric Advanced Life Support (PALS) Course, thanks in large part to the efforts of Dr. Leon Chemeides and others in promoting pediatric resuscitation.

PALS has become an integral part of the "alphabet soup" of courses often required of many physicians, nurses, respiratory care professionals, paramedics and emergency medical technicians. It provides a common language and approach in dealing with the critically ill child. It provides a mechanism for disseminating information in a period of increasingly rapid change, and it strives to provide evidence-based approaches in pediatric resuscitation. As of the publication of the 1997 edition of the *PALS Provider Manual*, over 50,000 had taken the course.

The purpose of this book is to encourage the learning and retention of the material presented in a PALS course. The authors have worked through the material paragraph by paragraph, creating questions about the information presented in that text. All of the answers are either direct quotes or paraphrases of the published materials. The primary purpose of *PALS Review* is to help you learn and review information by utilizing the Socratic method instead of reading a text. It will help you study and review information critical to improving the emergency care received by our children.

With this goal in mind, the text is written in question/answer format. The student receives immediate gratification with a correct answer. Misleading or confusing multiple-choice "foils" are *not* provided, thereby eliminating the risk of assimilating erroneous information. Another advantage of this format is that the student either knows or does not know the answer to a given question. This results in active learning, rather than the passive learning of studying multiple-choice questions. Active learning goes beyond the desire to pass an exam; when administering epinephrine to a child in cardiac arrest, you must know instantly that you need to push .01 mg/kg, and there will be nobody to ask you if you want to push a) 1mg, b) 0.1mg/kg, c) .01 mg/kg, or d) none of the above.

Questions may have answers without explanation. This is done to enhance ease of reading and rate of learning. Explanations often occur in a later question/answer. It may happen that upon reading an answer the reader may think – "Hmm, why is that?" or, "Are you sure?" If this happens to you, GO CHECK! Truly assimilating this information into a framework of knowledge absolutely requires further reading. Information learned as a response to seeking an answer to a particular question is much better retained than that passively read. Take advantage of this. Use *PALS Review* with your provider manual and preferred source texts handy and open or, if you are reviewing on a train, plane or camelback, mark the question for further investigation.

By definition, resuscitation courses are developed by consensus, and their texts must be produced on a given date. The dynamic knowledge base and clinical practice of medicine is not like that! The information taken as "correct" is that indicated by the 2000 Guidelines. New research and practice occasionally deviates from that which likely represents the "right" answer for test purposes. Refer to your most current sources of information and local authorities for direction on current practice.

PALS Review is designed to be used, not just read. It is an *interactive* text. Use a 3×5 card and cover the answer. Attempt all questions. A study method we strongly recommend is oral group study. The mechanics of this method are simple and no one ever appears stupid. One person holds *PALS Review*, with answers covered, and reads the question. Each person, including the reader says "Check!" when he or she has an answer in mind. After everyone has "checked" in, someone states his or her answer. If this answer is correct, on to the next one. If not, another person states his or her answer, or the answer can be read. Usually, the person who "checks" in first gets the first opportunity at stating the answer. If this person is being an answer-hog, then others can take turns. You can do it in teams. Try it—it's almost fun!

We welcome your comments, suggestions and criticism. Great effort has been made to verify these questions and answers. Please make us aware of any errata you find, as we hope to make continuous improvements in a subsequent edition and greatly appreciate any input concerning format, organization, content, presentation or about specific questions. We look forward to hearing from you.

Study hard and good luck!

Guy H. Haskell

TABLE OF CONTENTS

EMERGENCY MEDICAL SERVICES FOR CHILDREN

"The thing that impresses me the most about America is the way parents obey their children."
~ King Edward VII ~

"The functional survival of critically ill and injured children is influenced by the provision of timely and appropriate pediatric emergency care. This care includes a broad spectrum of services, from early identification of problems through pre-hospital, hospital, and rehabilitative care. Emergency Medical Services for Children (EMS-C) must therefore be integrated into emergency medical services (EMS) systems at state, regional and local levels. The specific needs of pediatric patients within the EMS system are now appreciated as a result of efforts by the pediatric and emergency medicine communities and projects funded through the U.S. Department of Health and Human Services, Health Services and Resources Administration, Maternal and Child Health Branch, in collaboration with the National Highway Traffic Safety Commission."

❍ **What is the key factor that will influence the functional survival of critically ill and injured children?**

The functional survival of critically ill and injured children is influenced by the provision of timely and appropriate pediatric emergency care.

❍ **What three areas of medical care are needed to optimize the functional outcome of an ill or injured child?**

Pre-hospital, hospital and rehabilitative care.

❍ **At which three levels of government should EMS-C be integrated into EMS?**

It must be integrated at the state, regional and local levels.

❍ **Which two agencies provide funding for education, training and research needed by EMS systems to treat pediatric patients?**

1. U.S. Dept. of Health and Human Services, Health Services and Resources Administration, Maternal and Child Health Branch
2. The National Highway Traffic Safety Administration

○   **Identify the four links in pediatric Chain of Survival.**

Injury prevention, early CPR, early access to EMS, and early advanced life support.

○   **List the two components of the first link (injury prevention) in the Chain of Survival for pediatric emergencies.**

Identification of problems and early intervention.

○   **In addition to health care professionals, who should be trained to recognize ill and injured children, provide first aid, activate EMS and be familiar with the resources for emergency care in their communities?**

Parents, caretakers and school personnel.

○   **List the minimal requirements of caretakers for children in regard to EMS-C.**

Caretakers of children must be able to recognize an emergency, initiate emergency care and rapidly call EMS.

○   **When does entry into the EMS system occur?**

Entry into the EMS system occurs when the rescuer or bystander calls local EMS and speaks with a dispatcher.

○   **What is considered the universal emergency access number?**

911.

○   **Is 911 access available in all communities?**

No, in 1991 only 60% of the total population and only 42% of the cities within the US could access emergency services by dialing 911.

○   **Describe the benefit of "enhanced 911" to a community.**

An enhanced 911-service enables immediate computerized identification of the telephone number and location of the caller so the dispatcher can send appropriate help regardless of the quality of the information provided by the caller.

○   **EMS dispatchers often provide a caller with pre-arrival directions. Who dictates what information is given to the caller?**

The information given callers varies widely and is controlled by local jurisdiction.

○   **Explain the advantages of using established dispatcher protocols when providing a caller with pre-arrival instructions.**

Use of dispatcher protocols will reduce the variability of information provided by dispatchers and ensure that succinct, accurate emergency information is provided to every caller in need of emergency assistance.

O   What percentage of EMS dispatchers is currently using protocols that outline pre-arrival instructions?

Less than 20% of all EMS dispatchers are using pre-arrival protocols.

O   What information should be included in pre-arrival instructions that are given to a caller in need of emergency care?

Instruction in pediatric CPR, relief of foreign-body airway obstruction, and essential first aid until EMS personnel arrive.

O   In the broad scope, "who" is actually the first link in the Chain of Survival?

The first link in the Chain of Survival is the general public.

O   Who is included in this "first link" as it applies to children?

Parents, caretakers, older siblings, and school personnel, who must be educated about the proper use of the EMS system.

O   What is the typical outcome of pediatric out-of-hospital asystolic cardiopulmonary arrest?

Typically, the child does not survive out-of-hospital cardiopulmonary arrest.

O   What types of equipment could be used as burn dressings in the pre-hospital pediatric equipment bag?

Burn dressings may include commercially available packs or clean sheets and dressings.

O   Approximately what percentage of EMS contacts in both rural and urban areas are children under 14 years of age?

10%.

O   What type of medical emergency results in the most contacts between EMS personnel and children between the ages of 5 and 14 years of age?

Trauma.

O   For children younger than five years of age, is the EMS system most frequently activated for trauma or medical illness?

Medical illness.

O   **Serious illness, including cardiopulmonary arrest, is most common in children of what age?**

2 years of age.

O   **A child-size ventilation bag used for resuscitation should have a reservoir of at least _____ml but no more than _____ml.**

450ml; 750ml.

O   **The use of a rigid cervical collar is often difficult in a small pediatric patient. Describe an alternative to this device.**

Cervical immobilization of small infants may be better achieved by the use of towels and tape rather than a rigid collar, which may not fit properly.

O   **If pre-hospital providers are expected to assess and stabilize children with critical illness and injuries, what must they have besides training and education?**

The proper equipment.

O   **What type of pediatric equipment is often missing from emergency vehicles?**

Too often pediatric intubation equipment, blood pressure cuffs, and vascular access catheters are missing from emergency vehicles.

O   **In addition to BLS equipment, list five items that should be included in a pre-hospital pediatric equipment bag for advanced life support units.**

Pediatric endotracheal tubes
Intraosseous needles
Pediatric laryngoscope
Pediatric Magill forceps
Pediatric stylettes for endotracheal tubes

O   **Using a conservative estimate, how many persons aged 0 to 19 years have permanent disabilities from traumatic brain injuries annually?**

Approximately 29,000.

O   **To assist pediatricians in the development of community and office readiness for emergency care, what agency has published guidelines for the role of the primary provider in EMS for children?**

The American Academy of Pediatrics.

RECOGNITION OF SHOCK AND RESPIRATORY FAILURE

"Nothing shocks me. I'm a scientist."
~ Harrison Ford as Indiana Jones ~

"Cardiopulmonary arrest in infants and children is rarely a sudden event. Instead, it is often the end result of progressive deterioration in respiratory and circulatory function. Regardless of the initiating event or disease process, the final common pathway in this deterioration is the development of cardiopulmonary failure and possible cardiopulmonary arrest. If pulseless cardiac arrest ensues, the outcome is dismal. Cardiopulmonary arrest can often be prevented if the clinician recognizes symptoms of respiratory failure of shock and promptly initiates therapy. This chapter presents guidelines for anticipating cardiopulmonary arrest in infants and children and for establishing priorities in care."

⭘ **What is cardiopulmonary arrest?**

Cardiopulmonary arrest refers to an apneic, pulseless state with cardiac standstill (asystole) or a dysrhythmia producing no cardiac output (ventricular fibrillation, ventricular tachycardia).

⭘ **Describe progression to non-traumatic cardiopulmonary arrest in children?**

Within the pediatric age group a cardiopulmonary arrest from a non-traumatic cause is rarely a sudden event. It occurs following an often-prolonged period of time during which a child's clinical condition deteriorates from a compensated state (respiratory distress or compensated circulatory failure) to a decompensated state (respiratory failure or decompensated shock) and finally to cardiopulmonary failure (global deficit in oxygenation, ventilation and perfusion). Once in cardiopulmonary failure, cardiopulmonary arrest is imminent.

⭘ **What is the outcome of cardiac arrest in infants and children?**

The outcome of cardiac arrest in children is dismal. Most (greater than 90%) of pediatric patients who present to an Emergency Department in asystole cannot be resuscitated. Only a very small percentage of those who survive are neurologically intact.

⭘ **What types of assessment skills must clinicians develop to prevent cardiopulmonary arrest in infants and children?**

It is important for clinicians caring for children to develop the cognitive and psychomotor skills necessary to recognize a child in shock or respiratory failure, preventing a complete cardiac arrest.

❍   **What cognitive skills must be developed in this regard?**

Important cognitive skills include the early recognition of respiratory failure, circulatory failure and cardiopulmonary failure.

❍   **What psychomotor skills must be learned in this regard?**

Important psychomotor skills include those necessary to initiate immediate management priorities: airway management, vascular access, fluid resuscitation, and treatment of dysrhythmias.

❍   **What are the six conditions requiring rapid cardiopulmonary assessment and potential cardiopulmonary support?**

Respiratory distress or failure
    Respiratory rate >60 breaths per minute
    Increased work of breathing
    Cyanosis or a decrease in oxyhemoglobin saturation
    Altered level of consciousness
Shock
    Heart rate: <5 years of age: <80 bpm or >180 bpm
                   >5 years of age: <60 bpm or >160 bpm
    Altered level of consciousness
Seizures
Fever with petechiae
Trauma
Burns involving >10% of body surface area

❍   **What are common causes of respiratory failure?**

Respiratory failure is most often the result of lower or upper airway obstructive or infectious processes in the lung or airway. Examples of these include pneumonia, bronchiolitis, asthma, croup, pharyngeal abscesses, epiglottitis, bacterial tracheitis and foreign body obstruction. These etiologies are usually associated with distress and increased work of breathing. Poor respiratory effort or hypoventilation without distress can also lead to respiratory failure. Examples of this include apnea in infants and hypoventilation following a head injury.

❍   **What is respiratory distress?**

Respiratory distress is a compensated state characterized by increased work of breathing. Adequate oxygenation and ventilation are maintained by the body's compensatory mechanisms and supplemental oxygen.

❍   **How does respiratory failure usually develop in infants and children?**

Respiratory failure is a decompensated state that usually follows a period of respiratory distress. A child in respiratory failure can no longer maintain adequate oxygenation and ventilation.

❍   **What are signs of respiratory distress (increased work of breathing) in a child or infant?**

Tachypnea, retractions, nasal flaring, grunting and tachycardia.

❍   **How is the diagnosis of respiratory failure made?**

Actual or impending respiratory failure is a clinical diagnosis based on an assessment of a child's inability to maintain oxygenation and ventilation.

❍   **What is the role of an arterial blood gas in making the diagnosis of respiratory failure?**

An arterial blood gas should be used to confirm the clinical suspicion of respiratory failure but not relied upon to make this diagnosis. The diagnosis of respiratory failure often must be made in settings where an ABG is not available. In addition, they must be interpreted within the context of the patient's present clinical state and past medical history.

❍   **What is shock?**

Shock is the clinical state of inadequate perfusion to meet the body's metabolic needs. Delivery of oxygen and important substrates (glucose) is impaired.

❍   **Does shock occur exclusively in low cardiac output states?**

Shock can occur in the setting of low, normal or increased cardiac output.

❍   **What is the difference between compensated and decompensated shock?**

In compensated shock, compensatory mechanisms (increased heart rate, increased peripheral vascular resistance) act to maintain adequate perfusion. Compensated shock is associated with an adequate blood pressure. Decompensated shock occurs when compensatory mechanisms have failed, perfusion is poor, and hypotension develops.

❍   **When does cardiopulmonary failure develop?**

As respiratory failure and decompensated shock progress, global deficits in oxygenation, ventilation and perfusion (or cardiopulmonary failure) develop. Inadequate oxygenation and perfusion results in insufficient delivery of oxygen and glucose to the tissues and inadequate clearance of the byproducts of metabolism.

❍   **What three factors determine oxygen delivery?**

Cardiac output, hemoglobin concentration and oxyhemoglobin saturation.

❍   **What are clinical signs of cardiopulmonary failure?**

Respiratory failure (cyanosis, pallor), altered level of consciousness (irritability, lethargy), and hypoperfusion (tachycardia, hypotonia, weak pulses, and prolonged capillary refill). Bradycardia, hypotension and hypoventilation are seen late in cardiopulmonary failure and are signs of an imminent cardiopulmonary arrest.

❍   **How does the normal respiratory rate vary in infants and children?**

A normal respiratory rate is inversely related to a child's age. It is normally fastest in the neonate and decreases throughout infancy and childhood.

❍   **What is the respiratory rate of an infant?**

30-60 breaths per minute.

❍   **What is the respiratory rate of a toddler?**

24-40 breaths per minute.

❍   **What is the respiratory rate of a preschooler?**

22-34 breaths per minute.

❍   **What is the respiratory rate for a school-age child?**

18-30 breaths per minute.

❍   **What is the respiratory rate of an adolescent?**

12-16 breaths per minute (same as an adult).

❍   **What is tidal volume?**

Tidal volume is the amount or volume of air that is moved with each breath. The total tidal volume increases with age (and size), but the tidal volume/kilogram remains constant throughout life.

❍   **How is tidal volume assessed?**

Tidal volume is best assessed clinically by observation of chest wall movement (chest rise) with ventilation and by listening to air movement throughout the lungs.

❍ **What is minute ventilation?**

Minute ventilation = tidal volume x respiratory rate.

❍ **How is minute ventilation compromised with respiratory distress or failure?**

Abnormalities in the respiratory rate, tidal volume or both will compromise minute ventilation. For example, a very slow respiratory rate (bradypnea) with an adequate tidal volume or a rapid respiratory rate (tachypnea) with a very small tidal volume will both result in abnormally low minute ventilation.

MV=RR X TV
MV $\downarrow$ when RR$\uparrow\uparrow$ as TV$\downarrow$
MV$\downarrow$ when RR$\downarrow$ as TV cannot $\uparrow$ to compensate

❍ **What should the initial assessment of respiratory function include?**

Respiratory rate (tachypnea, bradypnea, apnea), respiratory mechanics (retractions, nasal flaring, grunting, head bobbing), color of the skin and mucous membranes (cyanosis, pallor). Patients who are developing respiratory failure present with symptoms of hypoxia or hypercarbia (decreased level of consciousness, poor muscle tone, and cyanosis).

❍ **What is tachypnea?**

Tachypnea is an abnormally elevated respiratory rate. It is an early sign of respiratory distress in infants and children.

❍ **Is tachypnea always caused by respiratory problems?**

Tachypnea is a compensatory mechanism seen with metabolic acidosis, abdominal disorders and some toxic ingestion as well.

❍ **What is bradypnea?**

Bradypnea is an abnormally slow respiratory rate. An abnormally slow or decreasing respiratory rate is caused by fatigue and is an ominous sign of respiratory failure and decompensation.

❍ **What does the term "respiratory mechanics" mean?**

The mechanics of respiration is the work that goes into breathing: moving the chest wall and expanding the lungs. With respiratory distress either from upper or lower airway obstruction or from alveolar disease, the work of breathing is increased in an attempt to overcome underlying pathology.

○   **What are common signs of abnormal respiratory mechanics (increased work of breathing) seen in respiratory distress?**

Nasal flaring, grunting, intercostal, subcostal and suprasternal retractions, head bobbing, grunting, stridor, and prolonged expiration.

○   **What are "seesaw or rocky" respirations?**

Seesaw respirations or abdominal breathing is characterized by chest retractions accompanied by abdominal distention. It is an ineffective form of ventilation seen with severe respiratory distress and impending respiratory failure.

○   **What is grunting?**

Grunting is an ominous respiratory sound heard at the end of exhalation. It is an involuntary reflex in infants and is caused by exhalation against a prematurely closed glottis. Infants and children grunt in order to maintain or increase positive end expiratory pressure.

○   **With what conditions is grunting associated?**

Grunting is associated with conditions that result in hypoxia such as pulmonary edema and pneumonia.

○   **What is stridor?**

Stridor is a high-pitched inspiratory sound caused by extra-thoracic upper airway obstruction.

○   **What are common causes of upper airway obstructions in infants and young children that may present as stridor?**

Congenital anomalies (macroglossia, tracheomalacia, cysts, tumors or hemangiomas of the airway, vocal cord paralysis), infections (croup, epiglottitis, pharyngeal abscess, bacterial tracheitis), upper airway inflammation (allergy, post intubation), and esophageal or airway foreign body.

○   **What is wheezing?**

Wheezing is a sign of pathology in the lower airway usually caused by obstruction from inflammation or swelling at the bronchial or bronchiolar level. This type of obstruction causes air trapping and in addition to wheezing, prolonged expiration can also be appreciated on physical examination. On chest x-ray, the lungs look hyperinflated.

○   **What are common pediatric diagnoses that can cause prolonged expiration?**

Bronchiolitis, asthma, intrathoracic foreign body and rarely pulmonary edema.

❍ **Where should breath sounds be auscultated?**

Breath sounds should be auscultated over the anterior and posterior chest and in the axillae.

❍ **Describe normal breath sounds.**

Breath sounds should sound equal and easily heard bilaterally. A child's thin chest wall allows sound from the upper airway and the stomach to be transmitted throughout the chest.

❍ **During positive pressure ventilation how should the effectiveness of ventilation be assessed?**

Effective ventilation (the delivery of adequate tidal volume) should be assessed by both auscultation of breath sounds and observation of chest wall movement.

❍ **What should you observe regarding chest wall expansion?**

The chest wall should expand symmetrically with each breath.

❍ **What are the two primary causes of decreased bilateral chest expansion?**

Bilaterally decreased chest expansion may be caused by hypoventilation or lower or upper airway obstruction.

❍ **What are the possible causes of unilateral poor chest expansion?**

Unilateral poor chest expansion may result from a pneumo- or hemothorax, pleural effusion, mucous plug, foreign body in the right or left bronchial tree or endotracheal tube displaced in the right mainstem bronchus.

❍ **Is central cyanosis an early indicator of hypoxemia?**

Central cyanosis is a late sign of hypoxemia. It is generally associated with marked respiratory distress and/or respiratory failure.

❍ **Is central cyanosis always seen with hypoxemia?**

Cyanosis is not always a reliable indicator of hypoxemia. For cyanosis to be clinically apparent, 5 grams desaturated hemoglobin per deciliter of blood must be present. Therefore, cyanosis may not be observed in an anemic child who is hypoxic.

❍ **What is shock?**

Shock or circulatory failure is a clinical state characterized by inadequate perfusion of vital organs.

❍   **What are some consequences of circulatory failure?**

Inadequate delivery of important substrates (oxygen and glucose) and clearance of byproducts of metabolism results in anaerobic metabolism and lactic acidosis.

❍   **What is cardiac output?**

Cardiac output is the volume of blood ejected by the heart each minute. It is the product of the heart rate and stroke volume.

❍   **What is stroke volume?**

Stroke volume is the volume of blood ejected by the ventricles with each contraction.

❍   **What is arterial blood pressure?**

Arterial blood pressure is a reflection of both cardiac output and systemic vascular resistance.

❍   **What is the heart rate range of a newborn to 3 months?**

80 (with sleep)-160 beats per minute.

❍   **What is the heart rate range from 3 months to 2 years?**

75-190 beats per minute.

❍   **What is the heart rate range from 2 to 10 years?**

60-140 beats per minute.

❍   **What is the heart rate range >10 years?**

50-100 beats per minute.

❍   **What are the three etiologies of shock?**

Hypovolemic, distributive and cardiogenic.

❍   **What is the formula for estimating blood pressure in children 1-10 years of age (50th percentile)?**

90mm Hg + (child's age in years/2) mm Hg.

❍   **What is the formula for estimating the lower limits of systolic blood pressure in children 1-10 years of age (5th percentile)?**

70 mm Hg + (child's age in years/2) mm Hg.

❍   **What is hypovolemic shock?**

Hypovolemic shock, the most common form of shock in children, is caused by inadequate intravascular volume usually resulting from dehydration or hemorrhage.

❍   **What is distributive shock?**

Distributive shock is associated with loss of intravascular volume to extravascular tissues and systemic vasodilation. This form of shock is seen in the setting of anaphylaxis, sepsis and burns.

❍   **What is cardiogenic shock?**

Cardiogenic shock is caused by myocardial dysfunction and can occur with normal or increased intravascular volume. Cardiogenic shock occurs in the setting of congenital heart disease, dysrhythmias and infections of the heart muscles (myocarditis). Children who have required CPR or prolonged resuscitation should be assumed to have suffered some degree of myocardial dysfunction.

❍   **What is the difference between compensated and decompensated shock?**

Compensated and decompensated shocks occur in a continuum. In early or compensated shock, hypoperfusion of vital organs (decreased urine output, abnormal mental status) is present but compensatory mechanisms are sufficient to sustain adequate perfusion. Decompensated shock occurs when these compensatory mechanisms fail and organ perfusion worsens and hypotension develops.

❍   **How is shock related to cardiac output?**

Shock is usually associated with a decreased cardiac output (hypovolemia), however the hypoperfusion seen with sepsis and anaphylaxis can occur with an increased cardiac output.

❍   **What compensatory mechanisms occur when shock is associated with a low cardiac output state?**

Peripheral vascular resistance increases, the skin become cool and mottled and blood is diverted away from nonessential organs, such as the skin and mesentery. This redistribution of cardiac output and increased peripheral vascular resistance allows for an adequate blood pressure to be maintained.

❍   **What occurs in shock with high cardiac output?**

In a high cardiac output state such as anaphylaxis, low peripheral vascular resistance results in increased blood flow to the skin and periphery. The skin may appear pink and well perfused and peripheral pulses may be full or bounding.

❍   **Is sinus tachycardia commonly seen in infants and young children?**

Sinus tachycardia is an extremely common response to a variety of stimuli.

❍   **What are common causes of sinus tachycardia?**

Anxiety, pain, fever, hypoxia, hypercarbia, hypovolemia and cardiac disease.

❍   **Which compensatory mechanism maintains adequate cardiac output in the face of circulatory failure?**

Heart rate to a much greater extent than stroke volume influences cardiac output in infants and young children.

❍   **How does the heart rate respond to hypoxemia in neonates?**

Neonates develop bradycardia in response to hypoxemia.

❍   **What happens to the heart rate in older children in response to hypoxemia?**

The initial response to hypoxemia in older children is tachycardia. As hypoxemia persists, tachycardia is followed by bradycardia.

❍   **What is the significance of bradycardia in a child with cardiopulmonary failure?**

Bradycardia is a very serious sign of a decompensated state that immediately precedes a cardiopulmonary arrest.

❍   **What parameters determine a blood pressure?**

Cardiac output and peripheral vascular resistance.

❍   **What compensatory mechanisms come into play to maintain normal blood pressure despite falling cardiac output?**

Tachycardia, increased cardiac contractility (does not occur in young infants) and peripheral vasoconstriction.

❍   **What clinical state ensues when these compensatory mechanisms are no longer adequate?**

Decompensated shock usually accompanied by hypotension develops.

❍   **What is the significance of hypotension in a child with cardiopulmonary failure?**

Hypotension is a sign of endstage circulatory failure signaling depreciation of cardiovascular reserves and failure of compensatory mechanisms. It is rare but, when seen signifies an immanent cardiopulmonary arrest.

○ **How do normal blood pressures vary with age?**

The mean systolic blood pressure increases with age.

○ **What is the calculation for the circulating blood volume in neonates?**

85 ml/kg.

○ **What is the calculation for the circulatory blood volume in infants?**

80 ml/kg.

○ **What is the calculation for the circulatory blood volume in children?**

75 ml/kg.

○ **When is hypotension seen in children with acute blood loss?**

Hypotension is generally not observed until approximately 25% acute loss of circulating blood volume.

○ **What is the most important tool in assessing systemic perfusion in a child?**

The physical examination is of premiere importance in determining both the presence and degree of circulatory failure in children.

○ **What are the important components of the physical exam in assessing adequate perfusion in a child?**

Evaluation of central and peripheral pulses, skin perfusion, CNS perfusion and urine output.

○ **T/F: Heart rate and blood pressure are of limited value in the recognition of circulatory failure in children.**

True. Heart rate and blood pressure are of limited value in determining the presence and degree of circulatory failure.

○ **What is the significance of tachycardia in evaluating pediatric shock?**

Tachycardia is an early, nonspecific sign of anxiety and illness in children. Fever alone can cause significant tachycardia in some young patients. Most moderately and severely ill children will exhibit tachycardia.

❍ **When should tachycardia be taken seriously in children?**

Significant tachycardia (>160-180 beats per minute) should be taken seriously and monitored during treatment efforts and used to gauge of the success of resuscitative efforts.

❍ **What is the relationship between compensatory tachycardia and blood pressure?**

Because of compensatory tachycardia and peripheral vasoconstriction, the blood pressure is almost always found to be within the normal range in pediatric patients with progressing but still compensated circulatory failure.

❍ **Is blood pressure reliable for the diagnosis or estimate of degree of shock?**

Blood pressure alone is unreliable for the diagnosis or estimate of degree of shock.

❍ **What is the significance of hypotension in children?**

Hypotension in children is unusual, but when seen it is an ominous sign of decompensated circulatory failure.

❍ **How should the clinician evaluate circulatory failure in children?**

A carefully performed physical examination of end-organ perfusion as well as evaluation of vital signs will allow circulatory failure to be properly assessed.

❍ **What pulses should be evaluated in determining the degree of circulatory failure present in a child?**

The presence and the strength of both central (femoral) and peripheral (radial) pulses should be assessed.

❍ **As the cardiac output drops in the setting of hypovolemia, how do the peripheral pulses feel?**

The volume of the pulse seems diminished or thready. As hypoperfusion progresses, peripheral pulses may become absent.

❍ **What is the significance of the loss of central pulses in a child in cardiopulmonary failure?**

Loss of central pulses is a serious sign of an impending cardiopulmonary arrest.

❍ **What is the importance of an examination of the skin of a child who is in circulatory failure?**

Because of the high surface area to volume ratio in young children and infants, the skin is a relatively large organ as compared to adults. Decreased skin perfusion is a common and early sign of circulatory failure.

○ **What are signs of abnormal skin perfusion?**

Cooling of the skin peripherally, delayed capillary refill (>2 seconds), mottling, pallor and peripheral cyanosis. All of these signs (as well as decreased peripheral pulses) are seen in children and infants who are cold. Therefore these signs must be evaluated in the clinical and physical context of the patient. Infants and children should be kept in a warm environment in order to avoid confusion over the interpretation of poor skin signs.

○ **What are early signs of abnormal CNS perfusion?**

Signs of an abnormal mental status include confusion, irritability, lethargy, agitation and inappropriate behavior. An abnormal mental status in an infant or baby may be most easily assessed by observing the child's response to his parents, anxiety at parental separation and response to painful stimuli.

○ **What are clinical signs of severe and prolonged abnormal CNS perfusion?**

More profound change in mental status, loss of consciousness, abnormal muscle tones, seizures, and pupillary dilatation. A classification of a child's level of consciousness might include awake, responsive to voice, responsive to pain, and unresponsive.

○ **What is normal urinary output?**

Normal urinary output equals 1-2 ml/kg per hour.

○ **What three components make up a rapid cardiopulmonary assessment?**

Airway patency, adequacy of breathing and circulation (perfusion).

○ **What are the three classifications for pediatric airway patency?**

Patent, maintainable, and unmaintainable.

○ **What is the definition of a patent airway?**

No evidence of obstruction.

○ **What is the definition of a maintainable airway?**

A patient with a maintainable airway may benefit from head positioning, suctioning and/or the use of airway adjuncts. Harsh inspiratory sounds (stridor) originate from obstruction of the upper airway and should be noted while assessing the patency of the upper airway. A functional obstruction may exist because of abnormal positioning or secretions in the airway.

❍   **What is the definition of an unmaintainable airway?**

An airway unable to be maintained by simple maneuvers such as positioning or suctioning or one requiring immediate intervention such as assisted ventilation removal of foreign body, or intubation.

❍   **What specific parameters should be evaluated when assessing the adequacy of ventilation?**

Respiratory rate (too fast/too slow), air movement (quality and symmetry of breath sounds, chest expansion, chest wall movement) and abnormal sounds (snoring, stridor, wheezing), mechanics of breathing (retractions, grunting, nasal flaring) and skin color.

❍   **What parameters must be assessed in evaluating the degree of circulatory failure?**

Heart rate (tachycardia, bradycardia), blood pressure, peripheral and central pulses (presence and quality), skin perfusion (temperature, pallor, mottling, capillary refill), CNS perfusion (responsiveness, muscle tone, pupil size) and urine output.

❍   **What is the essence of a cardiopulmonary assessment?**

Cardiopulmonary assessment is a brief (30 second) examination of a critically ill child to detect deficits in oxygenation, ventilation and perfusion. It is not a complete physical examination. Assessments of any critically ill child must be repeated frequently as therapy is ongoing. Based on the cardiopulmonary assessment and resultant physiologic state, a child can be classified into one of six general groups.

❍   **What are the six stages of cardiopulmonary failure?**

Stable
Respiratory distress
Early circulatory failure
Respiratory failure
Late circulatory failure
Cardiopulmonary failure

❍   **What is respiratory distress?**

Increased work of breathing that may lead to or has the potential to become respiratory failure.

❍   **What is another name for early circulatory failure?**

Compensated shock.

❍   **Define late respiratory failure?**

A decompensated state marked by hypoxia and hypercarbia.

○ **Define late circulatory failure?**

Decompensated shock marked by hypotension.

○ **Define cardiopulmonary failure?**

Global deficits in oxygenation, ventilation and perfusion.

○ **Describe the management of a child who is in respiratory distress (potential respiratory failure).**

A child in respiratory distress without signs of respiratory failure should be allowed to assume a position of comfort (for example, remain in the parent's lap) and be given supplemental oxygen if needed. Generally these children benefit from monitoring of heart rate and oxygen saturation. A careful, unhurried physical exam should be conducted to look for the underlying cause of respiratory distress.

○ **Describe the approach to a child who is in respiratory failure.**

A child who presents with respiratory failure is in a decompensated state marked by hypoxemia and hypercarbia. In this condition, compensatory mechanisms have failed and inadequate oxygenation and ventilation have developed. The approach to a child in respiratory failure is to immediately establish a patent airway, begin adequate ventilation and administer 100% oxygen.

○ **Describe the approach to a child who is in compensated circulatory failure.**

A child in compensated circulatory failure is in a compensated clinical state marked by tachycardia, mild decreased urine output, mildly abnormal skin perfusion and mild signs of abnormal mental status. Vascular access should be obtained and a rapid blood sugar test may be helpful. A careful physical examination should be done to determine both the cause and degree of circulatory failure. Fluid resuscitation should follow.

○ **Describe the signs you expect to see in a child in decompensated shock.**

A child in late or decompensated shock presents with profound abnormalities in skin perfusion and mental status, tachycardia and oliguria. Peripheral pulses are absent, central pulses may be difficult to detect and hypotension may be present.

○ **What should your management be for this patient in decompensated shock?**

Attention should be paid to the adequacy of ventilation and airway patency in the setting of decompensated circulatory failure. This patient requires immediate and aggressive vascular access and fluid resuscitation.

❍ **Describe the signs you expect to see in cardiopulmonary failure.**

A child in cardiopulmonary failure presents with global deficits in oxygenation, ventilation and perfusion. This patient may be cyanotic, bradycardic, and severely hypoperfused. This very ominous constellation of clinical signs immediately precedes a complete cardiopulmonary arrest.

❍ **What should you do for this patient?**

A child who presents in cardiopulmonary failure requires the immediate establishment of a patent airway, initiation of assisted ventilation, administration of 100% oxygen and vascular access for fluid resuscitation and medications.

❍ **What are the causes of respiratory failure in a child who has suffered trauma?**

Respiratory failure may occur as a result of an injury to the brain, upper airway obstruction following trauma, injury to the lung or chest wall or even intra abdominal injury with restriction of movement of the diaphragm.

❍ **What traumatic chest injuries may result in respiratory failure?**

Pneumothorax, hemothorax, pulmonary contusion, flail chest.

❍ **What are the major causes of hemorrhagic shock?**

Trauma injuries to solid organs (liver or splenic laceration, hemothorax), fractures of large bones (femur fracture, pelvic fracture), and intracranial injury with hemorrhage or large soft tissue lacerations (scalp laceration) are all sources of significant blood loss.

❍ **What are some of the complications associated with burns in young children?**

Significant fluid loss through the burn and extravascular tissue occurs in children with burns in excess of 10% of the total body surface area. Inhalation injury from toxins and thermal injury may cause upper airway obstruction or respiratory failure and carbon monoxide poisoning.

❍ **What is epiglottitis?**

Epiglottitis is an invasive bacterial disease causing inflammation and edema of the epiglottis and a common cause of severe upper airway obstruction in children. Now it is more common in adults.

❍ **What are causes of acute deterioration during positive pressure ventilation?**

Endotracheal tube obstruction (mucus, blood, secretions), displacement (into the esophagus, pharynx or right main stem bronchus) tension pneumothorax, and mechanical equipment failure.

O   **How does respiratory distress or failure develop during seizures?**

Poor chest wall movement occurs during generalized tonic seizures leading to hypoventilation. Upper airway obstruction may be caused by tongue displacement and secretions. The effect of the above factors can be compounded by medications that cause respiratory depression. It is important to continuously monitor a child (especially heart rate and oxygen saturation) during, and following seizures.

O   **What are causes that predispose a child to stroke?**

Prematurity, Sickle Cell anemia, cyanotic congenital heart disease, coagulation disorders, trauma and arterial venous malformation.

O   **What data exist about the use of TPA for the treatment of stroke in neonates, infants and children?**

There is little data regarding the use of TPA for the treatment of strokes in patients less than 18 years of age. However, thrombolytic drugs may have some role in very select and unusual pediatric clinical entities.

O   **What are signs of increased intracranial pressure?**

Altered mental status (combativeness, irritability, somnolence), abnormal pupils (pupillary dilatation, lack of response to light, unequal size), and abnormal motor posturing.

O   **What are indications for intubation of a comatose child?**

Depressed mental status can be associated with hypoventilation (and the development of hypoxia and hypercarbia), loss of protective air reflexes and increased intracranial pressure. Intubation is indicated for oxygenation, control of intracranial hypertension (through mild hyperventilation) and protection of the airway.

O   **What is Cushing's triad?**

Cushing's triad is the combination of bradycardia, hypertension and irregular ineffective respiration. It is a late sign of increased intracranial pressure and impending herniation.

PEDIATRIC BASIC LIFE SUPPORT

"If you want to see what children can do, you must stop giving them things."
~ Norman Douglas ~

○ **T/F: Injury prevention is an important part of a community-wide effort to improve life support for infants and children.**

True.

○ **Who is usually present when a child has an out-of-hospital arrest?**

Parents or surrogates.

○ **Other than to parents, to whom should BLS courses be offered?**

Day care personnel, teachers, and coaches.

○ **T/F: Chronic illness is a risk factor for cardiopulmonary failure in children.**

True.

○ **What should the content of BLS courses include?**

Prevention, BLS techniques, and EMS system access.

○ **What group of professionals could take PALS courses?**

All pre-hospital and hospital personnel who care for infants and children.

○ **T/F: Primary cardiac arrest is the most common cause of death in young children.**

False. It is uncommon in children. Respiratory arrest usually precedes cardiac arrest.

○ **What percent of children present with ventricular fibrillation as a cause of pulseless arrest outside of the hospital?**

10-15%. Most are in asystole.

○ **Ventricular fibrillation is more likely in which patients?**

Children >10, submersion victims, those with congenital heart disease and in-hospital arrest.

❍   **What is the common primary cause of pulseless cardiac arrest?**

Injury or disease leading to respiratory or circulatory failure.

❍   **What percent of children survive pulseless out of hospital arrest?**

Survival is uncommon, about 10%.

❍   **In children, pre-hospital resuscitation should include what 3 things?**

Effective ventilation, oxygenation, and the prevention of cardiac arrest.

❍   **Cardiopulmonary arrest occurs predominately in which two pediatric age groups?**

Infants < 1year, and adolescents.

❍   **What are some of the common causes of cardiac arrest in infants?**

SIDS, injury (unintentional and intentional), ALTE, respiratory disease, airway obstruction, submersion, sepsis, and neurologic disease.

❍   **What is the most common cause of death in children >1 year of age?**

Injury.

❍   **What three principles of injury prevention should be emphasized?**

Passive injury prevention strategies
Specific instructions rather than general advice
Individual instruction reinforced by community-wide educational programs

❍   **Name the six most common types of severe childhood injuries.**

Motor vehicle passenger injuries
Pedestrian or bicycle injuries
Child maltreatment (abuse)
Submersion
Burns
Firearm injuries

❍   **Motor vehicle trauma accounts for what percent of all pediatric injuries and deaths?**

Almost 50%.

O   **What is the most important device to prevent pediatric motor vehicle injuries and deaths?**

A properly installed child restraint device.

O   **Do driver education classes reduce the incidence of collisions involving adolescents?**

No, these classes have increased the number of drivers without improving safety.

O   **What percent of adolescent motor vehicle fatalities involve alcohol?**

50%.

O   **What roadway improvements could help decrease pedestrian injuries?**

Adequate lighting, sidewalk construction, roadway barriers.

O   **What type of injury causes most bicycle related morbidity and mortality?**

Head injury.

O   **What percent of head injuries could bike helmets eliminate?**

85% of head injuries and 88% of brain injuries.

O   **What three things must helmet programs ensure to be successful?**

Acceptability, affordability and accessibility of helmets.

O   **What type of fence should enclose private swimming pools?**

5 feet high with self-latching, self-closing gate.

O   **What percent of fire-related deaths result from house fires?**

80%.

O   **What types of burns are common in children 4 years and younger?**

Smoke inhalation, scalds and electric burns.

O   **Smoke detectors can reduce the risk of death and severe injury by what percentage?**

90%.

❍   **How often should smoke detector batteries be changed?**

Twice a year.

❍   **T/F: Firearms are a leading cause of accidental death and injury in children.**

True.

❍   **Most guns found in the home used in unintentional shootings share what two characteristics?**

They are loaded and they are readily accessible.

❍   **T/F: The presence of a gun in the home is linked to adolescent suicide.**

True.

❍   **What are the key components of pediatric BLS?**

Sequential assessments and motor skills designed to support or restore effective ventilation and circulation.

❍   **What is the first step in BLS?**

Determine level of consciousness.

❍   **Why must unnecessary moving or shaking of the child be avoided?**

To prevent potential spinal cord injury.

❍   **T/F: An awake child with respiratory distress should be laid on the ground or on a stretcher.**

False. Children with partial airway obstruction will find the most comfortable position on their own.

❍   **If the child is conscious, when should EMS be activated?**

Immediately.

❍   **If the child is unconscious, how long should the rescuer provide BLS before activating EMS?**

1 minute. Most pediatric arrests are respiratory in origin, so one minute may be enough to restore ventilation and oxygenation or prevent respiratory arrest from progressing to cardiac arrest.

❍   **In an unconscious child, when should EMS be activated immediately?**

When two rescuers are present.

❍   **What should be done if trauma is suspected?**

Complete immobilization of the spine.

❍   **What are the most important components of BLS?**

Establishment and maintenance of a patent airway and support of adequate ventilation.

❍   **In an unconscious victim, what causes airway obstruction?**

Relaxation of muscles and posterior displacement of the tongue.

❍   **How can the airway be opened in an unconscious, apneic victim?**

Head tilt-chin lift.

❍   **How can the airway be opened in an unconscious, apneic victim if neck trauma is suspected?**

Jaw thrust with neck immobilized.

❍   **How is the head tilt-chin lift performed?**

One hand is used to tilt head and gently extend the neck. The index finger of the opposite hand lifts the chin outward.

❍   **After the airway is established, how does the rescuer assess breathing?**

Looks for rise and fall of the chest, listens for exhaled air, feels for exhaled airflow at the mouth.

❍   **What is the recovery position used for?**

When the victim is unconscious but has no evidence of trauma and is breathing effectively.

❍   **How is the victim moved into the recovery position?**

The head, torso, and shoulders are moved simultaneously so that the victim is on his or her side.

❍   **T/F: Rescue breathing is provided for all victims.**

False. Only those victims who have no spontaneous breathing.

❍ **In infants, how should rescue breaths be provided?**

By placing your mouth over the victim's nose and mouth.

❍ **How many breaths are supplied in rescue breathing?**

Two slow breaths, 1-1.5 seconds each separated by a pause to take a breath.

❍ **What is the purpose of the pause between rescue breaths?**

To maximize oxygen content.

❍ **T/F: Rescue breaths are the most important form of support for the non-breathing child.**
True.

❍ **How does the rescuer know if ventilation is not effective?**

The child's chest does not rise.

❍ **Why should breaths be delivered slowly?**

To minimize the pressure required for ventilation, and prevent gastric distension.

❍ **What is the most common cause of airway obstruction?**

Improper opening of the airway.

❍ **What should the rescuer do if ventilation is unsuccessful?**

Reposition the head in the midline, place a towel under the shoulders and consider progressively extending the neck, provided trauma is not suspected.

❍ **How may a second rescuer prevent gastric distension?**

By providing cricoid pressure.

❍ **What happens when cricoid pressure is performed?**

The trachea is displaced posteriorly compressing the esophagus against the vertebral column.

❍ **In a patient with a tracheostomy, how is air leakage prevented during rescue breathing?**

The victim's mouth and nose are sealed by the rescuer's hand or a tight fitting mask.

❍   **Are barrier devices effective for mouth-to-mouth ventilation?**

There are no adequate studies of the effectiveness of barrier devices.

❍   **When should the rescuer determine the need for chest compressions?**

After the airway is opened and two rescue breaths provided.

❍   **T/F: If the child is not breathing, chest compressions are usually required.**

True. Heart rate and stroke volume are probably not adequate if the child is not breathing.

❍   **What complications are common in children who receive CPR?**

None. Rib fractures in children are usually attributable to preceding trauma.

❍   **How long should the layperson spend looking for a pulse in a non-breathing child?**

No time. Laypersons often have difficulty recognizing pulses and should begin chest compressions immediately if the patient is not breathing or moving.

❍   **Where should the pulse be checked by health care professionals in infants?**

Brachial artery.

❍   **Where should the pulse be checked by health care professionals in children?**

The carotid artery should be used in children greater than 1 year of age.

❍   **If a pulse is present, how often should breaths be given?**

At a rate of 20 per minute.

❍   **If a pulse is present, when should EMS be activated?**

After 20 breaths or one minute.

❍   **What is the purpose of chest compressions?**

To circulate oxygen-containing blood to the vital organs.

❍   **What are the two theories for the mechanism of blood flow during chest compressions?**

Thoracic pump theory and cardiac pump theory.

❍   **To achieve optimal compressions, how should the child be positioned?**

Supine on a hard, flat surface.

O   **Where should you perform chest compressions on infants?**

Lower half of the sternum.

O   **How far should the infant's sternum be depressed during compressions?**

1/3 to 1/2 the depth of the chest.

O   **What should the rate of compressions be during infant CPR?**

At least 100 times per minute.

O   **What should the compression to ventilation ratio be?**

5:1.

O   **After what period of time should EMS be activated?**

20 cycles of CPR, about 1 minute.

O   **Children fall into what age-range for the purposes of BLS?**

Ages 1 year to 8 years.

O   **T/F: Compressions in children should be performed with the fingers.**

False. Compressions should be performed with the heel of the hand.

O   **What should the compression rate in children be?**

100 times per minute.

O   **What should the compression to ventilation ratio in children be?**

5:1.

O   **How often should the infant and child be reassessed?**

After 20 cycles of compressions and ventilation and every few minutes thereafter.

O   **How is airway patency maintained during compressions?**

The hand not doing compressions is used to maintain the head tilt.

O   **What information should be given to EMS?**

Location of the emergency
The telephone number from which the rescuer is calling
What happened
Number of victims
Nature of resuscitation

❍   **T/F: The majority of deaths from foreign body aspiration occur in children less than five years of age.**

True.

❍   **List common objects that can be aspirated.**

Toys, balloons, hot dogs, candies, nuts, and grapes.

❍   **What is a hallmark of foreign body aspiration?**

Sudden onset of respiratory distress.

❍   **When should infectious causes of airway obstruction be considered?**

When the child has a fever.

❍   **Name two infectious causes of airway obstruction.**

Croup and epiglottitis.

❍   **When should attempts to clear the airway be considered?**

When foreign-body aspiration is witnessed or strongly suspected
When the airway remains obstructed during rescue breathing attempts

❍   **T/F: Relief of airway obstruction should be attempted for all patients with foreign body aspiration.**

False. Only if signs of complete obstruction are observed.

❍   **What are the signs of complete airway obstruction?**

Ineffective cough, increased respiratory difficulty, development of cyanosis, loss of consciousness.

❍   **How does the Heimlich maneuver relieve foreign body obstruction?**

It increases intrathoracic pressure, creating an artificial cough which forces air and foreign bodies out of the airway.

❍   **For infants, what is the method by which complete foreign body obstruction is relieved?**

A combination of back blows and chest thrusts.

❍   **Why should the Heimlich maneuver not be performed on infants?**

There is a potential for liver injuries in these patients.

❍   **Why should blind finger sweeps be avoided?**

The foreign body may be pushed back into the airway.

❍   **How should back blows be delivered in an infant?**

Hold the infant face down, resting on forearm. The head should be lower than the trunk. Deliver back blows between scapulae with heel of hand.

❍   **How many back blows should be given?**

Five.

❍   **T/F: Chest thrusts in a choking infant are delivered in the same manner as chest compressions.**

True.

❍   **How long should the rescuer continue the series of back blows and chest thrusts?**

Until the object is expelled or the infant becomes unresponsive.

❍   **How are foreign bodies expelled in the conscious child?**

Abdominal thrusts while standing behind victim.

❍   **What should the protocol include if the child becomes unconscious?**

Attempt to visualize foreign body using tongue-jaw lift and remove it
Attempt rescue breathing
Straddle victim and perform abdominal thrusts
Repeat above steps until ventilation is successful

❍   **In the pediatric trauma victim, what may cause airway obstruction?**

Soft tissue swelling, blood, vomitus, or dental fragments.

❍   **What method should be used to open the airway in the trauma victim?**

Jaw-thrust ensuring that spinal stabilization has been achieved.

❍   Why is it difficult to maintain neutral c-spine position in infants and young children?

Prominent occiput predisposes the neck to slight flexion when the child is placed on a flat surface; this is why it is recommended to place a small towel under the shoulders to maintain the neck in neutral position.

AIRWAY AND VENTILATION

"I have found the best way to give advice to your children is to find out what they want and then advise them to do it."
~ Harry S Truman ~

"Respiratory problems are common in infants and children and are an important cause of in- and out-of-hospital cardiopulmonary arrest in the pediatric age group. Assessment and treatment decisions must be made quickly to prevent progression and deterioration to respiratory failure and cardiopulmonary arrest. If respiratory failure or respiratory arrest is promptly treated, intact survival of the child is likely. However, once respiratory arrest progresses to pulseless cardiac arrest, outcome is poor. Therefore, early recognition and effective management of respiratory problems are fundamental to pediatric advanced life support.

This chapter reviews the techniques and adjuncts used in airway management and the priorities of assessment and treatment of the infant and child with respiratory insufficiency or failure. Timely and appropriate use of these techniques and adjuncts is critical to the survival of the patient."

○ **Why should respiratory failure be treated promptly?**

To avoid progression to cardiac arrest which has a poor outcome in children.

○ **List the six ways the pediatric airway differs from the adult airway.**

The airway is smaller
The tongue is relatively larger
The larynx is more cephalad in position
The epiglottis is short, narrow and angled away from the trachea
The vocal cords attach lower anteriorly
In children less than 10 the narrowest portion of the airway is subglottic

○ **How can small amounts of edema effect the pediatric airway?**

They can significantly reduce airway diameter in children.

○ **Why should a straight laryngoscope blade be used in children?**

The high position of the larynx makes the angle between the tongue and glottis more acute.

O   **Should endotracheal tube size be based on the size of the glottic opening or the size of the cricoid ring?**

The cricoid ring, as this is the narrowest part of the trachea in children.

O   **How is airflow resistance related to airway radius?**

Inversely proportional to the fourth power of the airway radius during laminar flow (quiet breathing), and inversely proportional to the fifth power of airway radius during turbulent airflow.

O   **Why should the child with airway obstruction be kept calm?**

To prevent the generation of turbulent airflow.

O   **What structures normally support the lungs?**

The ribs and sternum.

O   **Why do the ribs fail to support the lungs adequately in the child?**

They are very compliant.

O   **What happens to functional residual capacity when respiratory effort is diminished?**

It is reduced.

O   **What is paradoxical chest movement?**

Sternal and intercostal retractions in response to airway obstruction during active inspiration.

O   **On what does tidal volume in infants and toddlers depend?**

Movement of the diaphragm.

O   **Why is the pediatric airway susceptible to dynamic collapse during airway obstruction?**

High compliance of the airway.

O   **How does PEEP improve airway exchange?**

By opposing the forces that cause dynamic airway collapse.

O   **Why do children have a high oxygen demand per kilogram?**

Their metabolic rate is high.

O   **Does hypoxemia occur more quickly in the child or adult in response to apnea?**

The child, secondary to high oxygen consumption.

O   **How does hypoxemia occur in response to respiratory distress?**

The disease process decreases lung compliance
The disease process increases airway resistance
The disease process interferes with oxygen or carbon dioxide exchange
Ventilation perfusion mismatch

O   **What are the two primary goals of emergency airway management?**

To anticipate and recognize respiratory problems
To support or replace functions that are reduced or lost

O   **Why should oxygen be administered to all seriously ill or injured patients?**

Oxygen delivery to tissues may be limited because of the arrest circulatory state.

O   **Why should oxygen be humidified?**

To prevent obstruction of small airways by dried secretions.

O   **Why should a heated humidification system be used?**

To prevent hypothermia in small patients.

O   **Why should children in respiratory distress be allowed to maintain a position of comfort?**

This position usually allows the maximal airway patency and minimizes respiratory effort.

O   **What does anxiety do to oxygen consumption?**

Increases it.

O   **What are alternative methods of providing oxygen supplementation?**

Blow-by or oxygen tent.

O   **What causes airway obstruction in a somnolent or unconscious child?**

Neck flexion, relaxation of the jaw, posterior displacement of the tongue, collapse of the hypopharynx.

○ **What can occur if breaths with a bag-valve-mask are not coordinated with the child's breathing efforts?**

Coughing, vomiting, laryngospasm, and gastric distension.

○ **Why is pulse oximetry an important technique for monitoring respiratory insufficiency?**

It provides continuous evaluation of arterial oxygen saturation.

○ **T/F: Pulse oximeters reflect the effectiveness of ventilation.**

False, they only evaluate level of oxygenation.

○ **When is the pulse oximeter's accuracy limited?**

In the presence of methemoglobinemia, carbon monoxide poisoning or in shock states.

○ **Why is the pulse oximeter not useful during shock or poor perfusion?**

It requires pulsatile blood flow to determine oxygen saturation.

○ **Where may the oximeter probe be placed if a signal is not detected at the fingertip?**

Ear lobe, nares, cheek, tongue and foot.

○ **What is an end tidal CO_2 detector used for?**

Allows for confirmation of endotracheal tube placement by percent of CO_2 found in exhaled air.

○ **What is the most accurate method of determining arterial oxygen concentration?**

Arterial blood gas.

○ **Why is a low flow oxygen delivery system insufficient to meet all inspiratory flow requirements?**

Because with low flow systems room air is entrained and mixed with the oxygen decreasing the concentration of oxygen to be inhaled by the patient.

○ **How is delivered oxygen concentration determined?**

By the patient's minute ventilation and gas flow delivery rate.

❍ **Which delivery system should be used in an emergency situation, high or low flow?**

High flow.

❍ **In a simple oxygen mask, what three things can reduce delivered oxygen concentration?**

If the patient's inspiratory flow rate is high, the mask is loose, or the oxygen flow into the mask is low.

❍ **What two valves does the nonrebreathing mask include to maximize inspired oxygen concentration?**

A valve that prevents entrainment of room air during inhalation
A valve that prevents flow of exhaled gas into the reservoir bag

❍ **What is the maximum inspired oxygen concentration achieved with a nonrebreather mask?**

95%.

❍ **What is an advantage of a face shield?**

Permits access to the face without interrupting oxygen flow.

❍ **What inspired oxygen concentration can be achieved with an oxygen hood?**

80-95%.

❍ **Is the nasal cannula a high flow or low flow system?**

Low flow.

❍ **What is the inspired oxygen concentration delivered by a nasal cannula?**

Cannot be easily or reliably determined, but is less than 50%.

❍ **What is the indication for use of an oral airway?**

In an unconscious child with airway obstruction after usual airway maneuvers have failed.

❍ **Why should an oral airway not be used in a conscious child?**

May stimulate gagging or vomiting.

○   **How is the appropriately sized oral airway chosen?**

Measure from the level of the central incisors, the bite block segment is parallel to the hard palate and the curved portion should reach the angle of the jaw.

○   **What is the appropriate length for a nasal airway?**

Distance from the tip of the nose to the tragus of the ear.

○   **What suction force is necessary to suction the airway of an infant or child?**

80-120 mmHg.

○   **What type of suction catheter should be used to suction secretions from an endotracheal tube?**

Flexible plastic suction catheter.

○   **Why should the heart rate be monitored during suctioning?**

Vagal stimulation and bradycardia can occur.

○   **What is the appropriate therapy once respiratory failure is recognized?**

Assisted ventilation.

○   **Why should the space under the mask used for ventilation be small?**

To decrease dead space and minimize rebreathing of exhaled gases.

○   **From where to where should the appropriately sized ventilation mask extend?**

The bridge of the nose to the cleft of the chin.

○   **When performing bag-valve-mask ventilation, why should pressure on the submental area be avoided?**

Can cause the tongue to be pushed into the posterior pharynx leading to obstruction or airway compression can occur.

○   **Where should the fingers be placed during BVM ventilation?**

On the jaw.

○   **What patient position is appropriate during BVM of infants and toddlers?**

Supine and head and neck in the neutral sniffing position.

O **What should be done if effective BVM ventilation cannot be achieved?**

Reposition head, make sure mask is snug, lift jaw, consider suctioning, ensure bag is functioning and connected to gas source.

O **What should be done if child is breathing spontaneously?**

Use 5 to 10 mmHg of continuous positive airway pressure (CPAP) to maintain airway patency.

O **How can gastric inflation be minimized in the unconscious child?**

Use appropriate sized equipment, only inflate the lungs with a volume necessary to initiate chest rise. Ventilate at an age appropriate rate, apply cricoid pressure.

O **How does cricoid pressure prevent gastric distension?**

Cricoid cartilage is displaced posteriorly compressing esophagus between the cricoid ring and the cervical spine.

O **What are the advantages of a self-inflating bag?**

Provides rapid means of ventilation in an emergency and does not require an oxygen source.

O **What does a self-inflating bag require to deliver higher than 80% oxygen?**

Oxygen reservoir.

O **T/F: Bags used for resuscitation should have no pop-off valve.**

True.

O **How can the pop-off valve be occluded in a self-inflating bag?**

Either by depressing the valve or twisting the valve into a closed position.

O **What can sudden decreases in lung compliance indicate?**

Right main bronchus intubation, obstructed endotracheal tube, and pneumothorax.

O **What minimum volume should resuscitation bags for full term infants have?**

450 ml.

❍   **T/F: Anesthesia ventilation systems require less experience to control than self-inflating bags.**

False, they require additional training to use effectively.

❍   **What must be adjusted to achieve ventilation with the anesthesia ventilation system?**

Fresh gas flow, outlet control valve, and proper facemask fit.

❍   **What happens if the fresh gas flow rate is increased?**

Decreased rebreathing of carbon dioxide, preventing hypercarbia.

❍   **Why can anesthesia ventilation systems be used during spontaneous respiration?**

No flow valves need to be opened.

❍   **What are some of the advantages of ventilation via an endotracheal tube?**

The airway is isolated
Potential for aspiration is reduced
Ventilations and chest compressions can be interposed efficiently
Inspiratory time and peek pressures can be controlled
PEEP can be delivered

❍   **What are six indications for intubation?**

1. Inadequate CNS control of ventilation
2. Loss of protective airway reflexes
3. Respiratory failure
4. Need for high ventilatory pressures or PEEP
5. Need for mechanical ventilatory support
6. Allows for stabilization of an airway that has the potential to deteriorate in transport or during special procedures at a hospital

❍   **What is the function of a Murphy eye on an endotracheal tube?**

Reduce the incidence of right upper lobe atelectasis and endotracheal tube obstruction.

❍   **When should a cuffed endotracheal tube be used?**

In children over 8 to 10 years old.

❍   **At what pressure should an air leak occur in the intubated patient?**

20 to 30 cm H_2O.

❍ **What does the absence of an air leak indicate?**

The cuff is inflated excessively, the ET tube is too large, or laryngospasm is occurring around the tube.

❍ **If visual inspection is used for choosing the endotracheal tube size, what part of the child's anatomy should be chosen for approximating the appropriate diameter?**

The width of a child's little fingernail.

❍ **What formula can be used to choose ET tube size in children over two?**

(Age [years]/4)+4.

❍ **What is the most accurate way of determining ET tube size?**

Using a length–based tape for weight estimate and then reading the appropriate tube size for that weight.

❍ **How can the ET tube size be used to estimate the depth of insertion of the tube?**

Internal diameter x 3 = depth of insertion (cm).

❍ **Which laryngoscope blade is preferred in infants and toddlers?**

Straight blade.

❍ **What equipment should be available prior to attempting intubation?**

Bag-valve-mask, oxygen, heart monitor, pulse oximeter, suction, laryngoscope, stylets, appropriate ET tube plus one size higher and lower, Magill forceps.

❍ **How should a stylet be placed in an ET tube?**

Lightly lubricated with tip inside distal end of ET tube.

❍ **What should be done if bradycardia occurs during intubation attempt?**

The procedure should be interrupted and the patient should be ventilated with 100% oxygen via bag-valve-mask.

❍ **Why and in whom should atropine be administered during intubation attempts?**

To prevent bradycardia in an infant or young child.

❍   **When should an intubation attempt be interrupted?**

If the patient develops hypoxemia, cyanosis, pallor, or decreased heart rate.

❍   **To directly visualize the glottis, what three structures must be aligned?**

The axes of the mouth, pharynx and trachea.

❍   **How should children less than two years old without trauma be placed for intubation?**

On a flat surface with the chin in sniffing position.

❍   **Why is orotracheal intubation preferred during resuscitation?**

It can be performed more rapidly than nasotracheal intubation and often with greater success.

❍   **Why should the blade not be inserted into the esophagus and withdrawn to visualize the epiglottis?**

This practice increases the risk of laryngeal trauma.

❍   **Where should the tip of the curved blade be placed?**

In the vallecula.

❍   **What is done with the tip of the straight blade?**

Used to lift the epiglottis to visualize the glottic opening.

❍   **From which direction should the endotracheal tube be inserted?**

From the right corner of the mouth.

❍   **How can an assistant make intubation easier?**

By displacing the right corner of the mouth to visualize the passage of the endotracheal tube, and applying cricoid pressure to facilitate visualization of the glottis.

❍   **Where is the black glottic marker on the endotracheal tube placed?**

At the level of or just below the vocal cords.

❍   **How is the position of the endotracheal tube assessed after intubation?**

Observation of symmetrical chest movement
Auscultation of equal breath sounds

Documentation of absent gurgling sounds over the stomach
Notation of end-tidal carbon dioxide level

O   **When can endotracheal carbon dioxide levels be low?**

In low cardiac output states.

O   **When should esophageal intubation be suspected?**

When the criteria for successful endotracheal intubation are not met, or there is abdominal distension during ventilation.

O   **How can proper position of the endotracheal tube be confirmed?**

Chest x-ray.

O   **What problems should be considered when intubation is confirmed but oxygenation or ventilation is inadequate?**

The endotracheal tube is too small
The pop off valve on the resuscitation bag is not depressed
A leak is present in the connections of the bag-valve device
Inadequate tidal volume is provided by the operator
Lack of lung expansion or lung collapse is occurring for other reasons

O   **How can displacement of the endotracheal tube be detected?**

By noting the distance marker number at the lips, by noting a deterioration in patient status, by use of end tidal CO_2 device, by decreased oxygen saturation, by clinical assessment that the tube is in the right mainstem (decreased breath sounds on the right versus the left) or by noting gurgling sounds in the stomach indicating esophageal displacement of the tube.

O   **Should esophageal obturator airways be used in children?**

No. They are too long and do not come in pediatric sizes.

O   **Why shouldn't oxygen powered breathing devices be used in children?**

High airway pressures may produce gastric distension or tension pneumothorax.

O   **When should tension pneumothorax be suspected?**

When any intubated patient deteriorates suddenly during positive pressure ventilation.

O   **What are the clinical signs of tension pneumothorax?**

Severe respiratory distress
Hyperresonance to percussion
Diminished breath sounds on the effected side
Deviation of the trachea and mediastinum away from the affected side

❍   **What is the treatment for tension pneumothorax?**

Immediate needle decompression.

❍   **For what clinical conditions might cricothyroidotomy be effective?**

Airway obstruction caused by foreign body, severe orofacial injuries, infection and laryngeal fracture.

❍   **What form of cricothyroidotomy should be performed by those without surgical training?**

Needle cricothyroidotomy.

❍   **What size needle should initially be placed through the cricothyroid membrane?**

20 gauge.

❍   **What signifies entry into the trachea?**

Aspiration of air.

❍   **What size cannula should eventually be placed?**

At least a 14 gauge.

❍   **How is the cannula connected to a bag valve device?**

Using a 3 mm endotracheal tube adapter.

❍   **What gas flow rate should be used for oxygenation in needle cricothyroidotomy?**

1 to 5 l/min (100cc/kg).

❍   **Patients with artificial airways are at risk for what problems?**

Loss of oxygen supply
Occlusion or kinking of the airway
Displacement of the airway

❍   **If a patient on a ventilator experiences a problem, what should be done?**

Patient should be manually ventilated with resuscitation bag using 100% oxygen.

○   **If the artificial airway is obstructed, what should be done first?**

Suction it with a large catheter.

○   **If the endotracheal tube is occluded and patency can't be restored, what should be done?**

Remove tube and ventilate with bag-valve -mask until reintubation.

○   **How are tracheostomy tubes held in place?**

By ties extending from the sides of the tube and fastened around the neck.

○   **What equipment should be kept at the bedside of a patient with a tracheostomy?**

A pair of scissors and a new tracheostomy tube.

○   **If recannulation of a patient's tracheostomy stoma cannot be accomplished, what should be done?**

Oral intubation, or bag- mask ventilation with gauze occluding the stoma, if there is no chest rise try placing a small mask over the stoma and performing mask to stoma ventilation using a bag valve device.

VASCULAR ACCESS

"After an access cover has been secured by 16 hold-down screws, it will be discovered that the gasket has been omitted."
"After the last of 16 mounting screws has been removed from an access cover, it will be discovered that the wrong access cover has been removed."
~ De La Lastra's Law ~

"Establishment of reliable vascular access is a crucial step in pediatric ALS. If vascular access is accomplished within the first minutes of resuscitation, infusion of medications and fluids is possible, and successful resuscitation may be more likely. Although the endotracheal tube may be used for emergency administration of some medications, intravenous or intraosseous access is preferred for drug delivery and is mandatory for the infusion of fluids, especially when cardiopulmonary compromise results from noncardiac causes, such as trauma or sepsis."

○ **What is the importance of vascular access in pediatric resuscitation?**

Establishing vascular access is the critical step necessary for drug and fluid administration for all patients in circulatory failure, respiratory failure, cardiopulmonary failure or cardiac arrest.

○ **T/F: Obtaining vascular access is one of the simplest tasks of pediatric emergency care.**

False. It is clearly one the most difficult technical aspects of pediatric emergency care.

○ **What is the preferred site for vascular access during CPR?**

Venous access during CPR should be rapidly established in the largest possible vein without interruption of CPR or airway management.

○ **Is peripheral access acceptable in pediatric resuscitation?**

Yes. A rapidly established peripheral venous line is an acceptable site for fluid and drug administration.

○ **What should you do if you cannot establish peripheral access quickly during resuscitation?**

If peripheral access cannot be established within the first several minutes of resuscitation, an alternative route must be pursued.

❍   **What are acceptable sites for peripheral access during resuscitation?**

Peripheral IVs can be started in the arms, hands, legs or feet. Very small veins of the hands and feet are extremely difficult to cannulate in the setting of circulatory collapse and larger peripheral veins should be chosen (saphenous, antecubital fossa). Scalp veins (relatively straight and visible) may be an alternative in a young baby who requires fluid resuscitation only. Scalp IVs are generally impractical in a child requiring airway management.

❍   **What is the value of intraosseous access during pediatric resuscitation?**

Intraosseous access is an extremely valuable alternative to peripheral access in infants and young children. The intraosseous route can be used for the administration of virtually all drugs, fluid and blood products that might be lifesaving.

❍   **Under what circumstances should a central venous line be placed during pediatric resuscitation?**

A central venous line is a very desirable alternative to peripheral access in a child requiring ongoing resuscitation, but requires a skilled provider and is often more time consuming than peripheral or IO access.

❍   **What is the most frequently used site for central venous cannulation and why?**

The femoral vein is the most frequently used central vein because it is large, anatomically reliable and can be cannulated without interrupting resuscitation.

❍   **T/F: A central line should always be attempted when the proper equipment is available.**

False. An experienced practitioner should attempt a central line.

❍   **T/F: If a central line will soon be available, delay administering medications and fluids until it is established.**

False, establishment of a central line should not delay the administration of resuscitation medications and fluids.

❍   **What equipment is important for the safe administration of fluids and medications in infants and young children?**

Infusion pumps or volume limiting devices such as minidrip chambers (if pumps are not available) should be used to safely administer fluid boluses and medication infusions in infants and young children.

❍   **During CPR in young children what strategy should be followed for establishing vascular access?**

In general, intraosseous access should be established following three attempts at peripheral vascular access (approximately 90 seconds).

❍   **Is intraosseous access appropriate for children older than 6 years of age?**

Yes. The PALS 2000 guidelines have removed the upper age limit for intraosseous access. However, keep in mind that intraosseous access becomes progressively more difficult in older children. If intraosseous access must be attempted in older patients, needles with threaded tips and alternative sites (iliac crest) should be considered to ensure success. In addition, peripheral vascular access is likely to be successful in older children.

❍   **Does a particular site insure more rapid delivery of medications to the central circulation during CPR?**

There is no significant difference between peripheral, intraosseous or central access with respect to onset of drug action or peak drug levels.

❍   **What should always be done immediately following a bolus infusion?**

It is important to follow medication delivery with a 5 cc fluid bolus to flush the drug to the central circulation.

❍   **What is the most important factor in determining route of intravenous access?**

Rapid access should be sought using the technique with which the medical personnel are most familiar.

❍   **What is the indication for ETT medication administration?**

If IV/IO access cannot be established within 3-5 minutes, the ETT is an important route for administration of medications.

❍   **What medications can be infused through the ETT?**

Lidocaine, epinephrine, atropine, naloxone (L.E.A.N.).

❍   **What veins should be attempted for peripheral access during resuscitation?**

In the setting of circulatory collapse, veins are difficult to see or palpate. Veins that are anatomically reliable are good choices for a "blind stick". Two of these are the greater saphenous (medial surface of the ankle) and the median cubital (antecubital fossa of elbow).

❍   **When should scalp veins be used?**

Scalp veins are usually straight and easy to see in infants, but are impractical during resuscitation requiring airway management. Scalp veins are of value when only fluids and medications are needed or in postresuscitation treatment as a temporizing measure until definitive access is achieved.

❍   **What are complications of peripheral IVs?**

Complications of peripheral IVs are relatively rare but include cellulitis, thrombosis, and infiltration.

❍   **What are the most common causes of sclerosis and skin sloughing following IV cannulation?**

Sclerosis and skin sloughing are most often related to necrotizing medications such as calcium and dextrose.

❍   **What two devices are commonly used for peripheral access?**

Over-the-needle catheters and butterfly needles.

❍   **Which is preferred?**

Over-the-needle catheters. These are either straight catheters with a clear hub or have butterfly grips and are attached to tubing. Some of these can be converted to a central catheter.

❍   **What value are butterfly needles?**

Butterfly needles are straight steel needles that are inserted into the vein. They are often used for scalp veins but are more prone to lacerate the vein and infiltrate than a catheter. Generally, butterfly needles are used for short-term access until definitive access can be established.

❍   **What is the technique for establishing peripheral access?**

Practice universal precautions
Identify and immobilize the site
Apply a proximal tourniquet
Prep the overlying skin
Puncture the skin and vein with the needle and catheter. If the skin is tough, a separate skin puncture that does not puncture the vein can be made first by pulling the skin to the side of the vein and puncturing it with a separate slightly larger needle.
Release the skin and pass the catheter and needle through the puncture site and into the vein.
Holding the needle bevel down may be helpful

Observe blood return and pass the catheter over the needle
Remove the needle
Remove the tourniquet
Secure the catheter and begin infusion

O **Describe the differences in this technique when inserting a butterfly needle into a scalp vein.**

A rubber band around the head should be used in place of a tourniquet
Flush the butterfly and tubing with normal saline
Introduce the needle through the skin and slowly advance it into the vein until blood
   flushes back into the tubing
Remove the rubber band tourniquet
Connect a syringe of saline and flush a small volume of fluid to evaluate the site for
   infiltration

O **What is the role of intraosseous access during pediatric resuscitation?**

Intraosseous access is an extremely valuable alternative to peripheral access in infants and young children. The intraosseous route can be used for the administration of virtually all drugs, fluid and blood products that might be lifesaving during the course of a particular resuscitation.

O **Is there any evidence to suggest that a particular technique or site insures more rapid delivery of resuscitation and medications to the central circulation?**

There is no data that suggests that there is a significant difference between peripheral intraosseous or central access with respect to onset of drug action or peak-drug levels. Clinicians should attempt rapid access using the technique with which they are most comfortable.

O **What are complications of intraosseous cannulation?**

Tibial fracture, compartment syndrome, osteomyelitis and skin cellulitis.

O **What is the incidence of intraosseous complications?**

Serious clinically significant complications following intraosseous access are in the range of 1%.

O **What are the different types of intraosseous needles?**

Jamshidi bone marrow aspiration needles are among the first needles to be used to cannulate the bone marrow for resuscitation purposes. These can be used in an emergency if alternatives are unavailable. The other kind of commonly available intraosseous needle is a specially designed needle for intraosseous infusions.

❍   **What site is generally recommended for the placement of an intraosseous needle?**

The anteromedial tibial surface 2-3 cm. below the tibial tuberosity is the preferred site for intraosseous needle placement in children.

❍   **Describe the technique for placement of an intraosseous line.**

Identify the tibial plateau located on the anterior medial surface of the tibia just distal to the tibial tuberosity
Cleanse the overlying skin
Inspect the needle apparatus to be sure that the stylette extends below the needle
Immobilize the leg so that the tibial plateau is approximately horizontal to the bed (do not place your hand underneath the patient's leg!)
Insert the needle through the skin and soft tissue advancing it until periosteum is contacted
Advance the needle through the bony cortex so that the needle is perpendicular to the patient's leg. Advancing the needle should be done with controlled pressure. Gently rotating the needle may be helpful
Advance the needle until a change in resistance is felt
Unscrew the needle cap and attempt to aspirate marrow
Ensure that the needle is secure in the bone
Stabilize the intraosseous needle
Begin infusion of 10-20cc. of normal saline
Inspect the intraosseous site again for signs of infiltration

❍   **What are signs that intraosseous insertion is successful?**

The subjective sense of a decrease in resistance as the needle passes through the cortex and into the marrow
The needle is stable in the bone and remains upright without support
Marrow can be aspirated through the needle into a syringe
Infusion through the needle does not show evidence of infiltration of the soft tissue

❍   **What should you do if you are unsuccessful on your first attempt at intraosseous cannulation?**

This same site cannot be used again. The procedure should be attempted on the other leg.

❍   **What are two advantages of central venous access in resuscitation?**

Central venous access allows rapid delivery of drugs to the central circulation and also allows monitoring of central venous pressures.

❍   **Are central venous lines, peripheral lines, or intraosseous lines more subject to complications?**

Central lines are clearly associated with more serious complications then peripheral or intraosseous lines. The specific complications are a function of the site of the central line.

❍ **What complications are associated with all central lines?**

All central lines are associated with increased risk of local and systemic infection, bleeding, phlebitis, thrombosis, catheter fragment and embolism.

❍ **What complications are associated with central lines in the neck?**

Central lines in the neck are associated with additional complications of pneumothorax, hydrothorax, and hemothorax.

❍ **Are complications more common in central lines in children or adults?**

In general complications of central venous access are more common in younger patients, therefore, a central line in children should be placed by an experienced clinician.

❍ **What general techniques have been employed in achieving central venous access in children?**

Both through the needle and over the needle catheter placement has been used to establish central venous access in children.

❍ **What are the hazards of through-the-needle catheter placement?**

The catheter can be sheared off by the sharp needle during placement of a through the needle catheter.

❍ **When does catheter shear usually occur when placing a through-the-needle catheter?**

This usually occurs when resistance is encountered as the catheter is advanced and the catheter has been withdrawn through the needle.

❍ **What can be done to reduce the possibility of catheter shear?**

The catheter should never be withdrawn through the needle. The entire catheter and needle apparatus should be withdrawn as a unit to prevent the complications of catheter shearing.

❍ **What is the most commonly used technique for central venous access in children?**

The Seldinger technique, which uses a guide wire to establish catheter placement, is the most commonly used technique for placement of central lines in children.

O **Describe the process by which a central line is placed using the Seldinger technique?**

A finer needle is used to locate the vein. Once blood flow is established through the needle, a guide wire is threaded through the needle and into the vessel. The finer needle can be removed and a catheter slid over the guide wire and into the vessel.

O **What is the most frequently used site for central venous access and why?**

The femoral vein is most frequently used because of its lower incidence of complications than central access in the neck, as well as the ease of starting a line far from the head and neck, which would interfere with CPR and airway management.

AA What are two commonly used veins in the neck for central venous access?

The internal jugular and the subclavian vein.

O **What are the advantages of cannulating the external jugular vein?**

The external jugular vein is a superficial vessel that is easily visible. When cannulated there is a large IV that allows rapid infusion of drugs and medication. An external jugular line on occasion can be converted to a central line, but this is at times impossible because of the acute angle of the external jugular into the subclavian vein.

O **What factor limits the use of the external jugular vein for vascular access in a child undergoing resuscitation?**

Successful cannulation of the external jugular vein requires positioning of the patient's head rotated away from the site and occasionally placement of the patient in Trendelenburg. These maneuvers may interfere with airway management and make placement of this line in patients requiring airway management impractical.

O **Why is the right internal jugular vein preferred for central venous access?**

The right internal jugular vein is preferred over the left because right-sided access is associated with a lower risk of pneumothorax and thoracic duct damage.

O **Describe the technique of femoral vein access?**

Position the leg with slight external rotation
Identify the femoral vein by palpation of the femoral artery just lateral to the femoral
   vein, or by finding the midpoint between the anterior/superior iliac spine and the pubic
   symphysis
Locate the vessel with a finer needle about 2 cm below the inguinal ligament. Once blood
   flow is established through the needle into a syringe disconnect the syringe and place
   your thumb over the hub of the needle

Introduce and advance the guide wire through the needle. Never advance a catheter or
　　guide wire against resistance
Remove the needle. Nick the skin with a scalpel to widen the opening for catheter
　　passage.
Advance a catheter over the wire into the femoral vein. The guide wire is then removed
Secure the catheter and get a chest x-ray to verify line placement

O   **Describe the technique for external jugular venous access.**

Position the child in Trendelenburg with the head turned away from the side to be
　　accessed. The right side is generally preferred for access
Identify the external jugular vein
Occlude the vein above the clavicle by gentle pressure with either a finger or a tongue
　　depressor Insert an over the needle catheter into the vein
Remove the needle and secure the catheter
Infrequently, central venous access is attempted through this route using the Seldinger
　　technique described above.

O   **Describe the technique for internal jugular vein access?**

Hyper-extend the patient's neck by placing a towel between the patient's shoulders
Place the child in Trendelenburg rotating the head slightly away from the site of access.
　　The right side is preferred for access
Identify the sternocleidomastoid and the clavicle
Advance the needle using the landmarks for either an anterior central or posterior
　　approach
When blood is flowing freely from the needle into a syringe, disconnect the syringe and
　　place your thumb over the hub of the needle
Introduce a guide wire, nick the skin, pass a dilator over the wire to widen the opening
　　being sure to always have a portion of the wire in your hand and then complete
　　placement of the central line using a Seldinger technique described above

O   **What is the technique for subclavian central venous access?**

Hyper-extend the patient's neck by placing a towel rolled beneath their shoulders and
　　place the child in Trendelenburg with the head turned slightly away from the side to be
　　accessed. The right side is preferred
Identify the juncture of the middle and medial thirds of the clavicle
Introduce a finer needle just under the clavicle at the junction of the middle and medial
　　thirds of the clavicle. When blood is freely flowing from the needle into a syringe,
　　disconnect the syringe, cover the hub with your thumb and introduce a guide wire
　　through the needle Continue as noted above

O   **What additional practices must be employed when starting central venous
access in children?**

Always practice universal precautions
Carefully cleanse the skin before access is attempted

Consider local anesthesia for patients who are conscious

❍   **Who should perform central venous access in children?**

Central venous line placement should only be performed by experienced practitioners. This is especially true for internal jugular and subclavian access in the neck.

❍   **Where is the saphenous vein most easily palpated?**

The saphenous vein is a long vein that courses down the leg and is most easily seen and palpated anterior to the medial malleolus.

❍   **What two methods are used for cannulating the saphenous vein?**

It can be cannulated by either a blind stick or through a cut-down when other forms of access are not achieved.

❍   **T/F: Saphenous vein cutdown is an quick and excellent technique for achieving vascular access in children in cardiopulmonary arrest when other methods are unsuccessful.**

False. Saphenous vein access is a time consuming procedure that is especially difficult in patients with low cardiac output, making it an impractical site for initial vascular access in children who have suffered a cardiopulmonary arrest.

❍   **Describe the technique for saphenous vein cut-down.**

Identify site of the saphenous vein anterior to the medial malleolus
Make a 2 cm incision superior and anterior to the medial malleolus
Carefully dissect subcutaneous tissue to expose the superficial fascia
In a direction parallel to the long access of the tibia, pierce and gently open the
    superficial fascia
Pass the tips of a hemostat into the incision and to the bone opening the hemostat into the
    incision site
The saphenous vein should be identified
Place ligature around the distal part of the vein
Place and do not tie a ligature around the proximal end of the vein
Pierce a small hole through the upper most vessel wall and pass a catheter through this
    small incision (venotomy)
Tie the proximal ligature around the vein and catheter
Remove the tourniquet
Secure the catheter in place

❍   **What are advantages to arterial access?**

Arterial catheters are extremely useful in monitoring blood pressure and for ease in blood sampling.

○   **What are complications of arterial catheters?**

Infection, embolus, arterial thrombus, ischemia or damaged to the effective limb.

○   **What is the most common complication of radial artery catheterization in children?**

Highest risk of radial artery occlusion includes patient age less than 5 years, access obtained through cut-down, and indwelling catheter of more than 4 days.

○   **What are acceptable sites for arterial catheterization?**

Radial, brachial, axillary, femoral, dorsalis pedis, and posterior tibial arteries.

○   **Which two of the these are preferred?**

Radial and femoral artery.

○   **What is the Allen test?**

The Allen test is used to assess adequacy of arterial blood flow through the ulnar artery prior to insertion of a radioarterial line.

FLUID THERAPY AND MEDICATIONS

*"The reason grandparents and grandchildren get along so well is that
they have a common enemy."*
~ Sam Levenson ~

*"This chapter reviews the pharmacology of drugs essential for resuscitation and
stabilization of infants and children and includes a discussion of fluid therapy and acid-
base balance. Therapeutic considerations, indications, doses, routes of administration,
precautions, and clinically recommended available forms of medications used in the
resuscitation and advanced life support of infants and children are also presented."*

❍ **What are the three major objectives of fluid administration during
resuscitation?**

Restore circulating volume for hypovolemic shock
Restore oxygen-carrying capacity for hemorrhagic shock
Correct metabolic acidosis

❍ **What are two causes of acid-base imbalance?**

Respiratory failure
Circulatory failure

❍ **What are five objectives of medication administration during resuscitation?**

Enhance coronary and cerebral perfusion during CPR
Stimulate more forceful cardiac contractions
Increase the heart rate
Correct metabolic acidosis
Suppress ventricular dysrhythmias

❍ **What is the most common cause of shock in children?**

Hypovolemic shock.

❍ **What are three causes of (volume loss) hypovolemic shock?**

GI losses through vomiting and diarrhea

Diabetic ketoacidosis through increased urination (diuresis)
Trauma

○   **What kind of shock is caused by peripheral vasodilatation resulting in venous pooling of blood and a decrease of blood returning to the central circulation?**

Neurogenic shock.

○   **What types of shock result from both vasodilatation and increased capillary permeability causing plasma losses out of the vascular space and into the interstitium caused?**

Septic shock
Anaphylactic shock

○   **What is shock resulting from inadequate heart (pump) function called?**

Cardiogenic shock.

○   **What are the three types of fluids that may be used in volume resuscitation in children with hypovolemic shock?**

Isotonic crystalloid
Colloid
Blood products

○   **Two types of crystalloid are?**

Normal saline
Lactated Ringers

○   **Why is it necessary to use large quantities of crystalloid to restore intravascular volume?**

Because over time only about one fourth of the crystalloid infused remains in the intravascular space.

○   **Name three types of colloid solutions.**

Albumin 5%
Fresh frozen plasma
Synthetics

○   **Name two examples of synthetic colloid preparations.**

Hetastarch
Dextran

❍ **T/F: Blood products are considered the first choice treatment for the management of hypovolemia.**

False. Crystalloids should be tried first.

❍ **When is blood considered the ideal fluid replacement in volume loss?**

When trauma victims in hypovolemic shock do not respond to crystalloid management or trauma patients present in decompensated shock.

❍ **What is the blood type that may be administered without crossmatch?**

O-negative.

❍ **Rapid infusion of cold blood or blood products containing citrate in large volumes may result in what two major complications?**

Hypothermia
Hypocalcemia

❍ **When is volume therapy indicated?**

When the child demonstrates signs and symptoms of shock.

❍ **What are five significant signs of hypovolemic shock in a child?**

Tachycardia
Pale, mottled, cool skin
Delayed capillary refill
Diminished peripheral pulses
Altered mental status

❍ **T/F: Optimum vascular access in a child requires only one large bore peripheral line.**

False. At least two are required.

❍ **What is the fluid bolus dose of crystalloid for the management of the symptomatic hypovolemic child?**

20ml/kg IV in less than 20 minutes.

❍ **How many times may fluid boluses of crystalloid be repeated during the first hour to manage volume losses in a hypovolemic child?**

Twice.

○   **T/F: It is more efficient to administer bolus fluid infusions by IV push with a syringe than with an IV drip.**

True. In children the volumes are smaller than in adults, and the fluids can be pushed faster.

○   **T/F: A child in septic shock may require 60 to 80ml/kg during the first hour of resuscitation.**

True.

○   **What should you do following each volume bolus?**

Reassess perfusion status of the child. Evaluate for effectiveness of therapy.

○   **T/F: Large volumes of dextrose containing solutions are particularly useful during volume resuscitation.**

False. They can be harmful because of their hypertonic effects.

○   **What is a chemical substance that helps to correct pH (acidity/alkalinity) imbalances of plasma called?**

A buffer.

○   **What is the most important (fastest) buffer system?**

The bicarbonate buffer system.

○   **To what does pH refer?**

The hydrogen concentration in the plasma.

○   **How is carbonic acid (H_2CO_3) formed?**

HCO_3 + H ion = H_2CO_3.

○   **What does a low pH measurement indicate?**

An increase in plasma acidity.

○   **What is the normal pH range?**

7.35 - 7.45.

○   **What is the normal $PaCO_2$ range?**

35 - 45mmHg.

❍ **What happens to the pH if the $PaCO_2$ rises?**

The pH will go down indicating increased plasma acidity.

❍ **Causes of reduced pH, i.e. respiratory verses metabolic, can be determined by referring to the $PaCO_2$ and HCO_3. What cause (respiratory or metabolic) would an elevation in $PaCO_2$ indicate?**

A respiratory component.

❍ **As $PaCO_2$ rises what system will compensate for this increase in CO_2?**

The respiratory system will compensate by increasing rate and tidal volume.

❍ **What is the normal ratio of base to acid?**

20:1.

❍ **What four components must be evaluated in order to interpret arterial blood gases?**

pH
$PaCO_2$
HCO_3
PO_2

❍ **ABG indicates a pH of 7.22, $PaCO_2$ of 40mmHg and HCO_3 of 8. Is this a metabolic acidemia or a respiratory acidemia?**

This is a metabolic acidemia because the $PaCO_2$ is normal and the HCO_3 is reduced.

❍ **An 18-month-old 10kg baby has an ABG as follows: pH 7.20 $PaCO_2$ 60mmHg HCO_3 24. Is this a metabolic or a respiratory problem?**

This is a respiratory acidemia because the $PaCO_2$ is elevated and the HCO_3 is normal.

❍ **What would be the appropriate management of a patient with a respiratory acidemia?**

Adequate oxygenation and appropriate ventilation.

❍ **What would be the appropriate management of a patient with a metabolic acidemia secondary to poor perfusion?**

Correct the perfusion problem (Volume, Pump, and Container) as required.

❍ **How do you determine a base deficit in the setting of a metabolic acidemia?**

Calculate the difference between the predicted pH (7.40) and the measured pH
Multiply the difference by 67 (constant)
This will give you the patient's base deficit

Example: Measured pH 7.18
Predicted pH 7.40
Difference: -0.22

-0.22 x 67 = -14.7 Base Deficit

○ **How do you calculate the appropriate NaHCO₃ to correct the base deficit for an 18kg baby in metabolic acidosis (pH 7.18)?**

Multiply the BASE DEFICIT x Pt. kg. wt. x 0.3 (constant) = NaHCO₃ dose (mEq)
Example: 14.7 Base Deficit x 18kg. x 0.3 = 79mEq NaHCO₃

○ **What is the ideal management for the correction of acidosis?**

Restoration of adequate systemic perfusion and effective ventilation.

○ **What is the preferred route for drug administration?**

The intravenous route.

○ **What two other routes are recommended for the administration of some drugs if the intravenous route is not available?**

The endotracheal route
The intraosseous route

○ **What drugs are indicated as approved for the endotracheal route of administration?**

Lidocaine
Epinephrine
Atropine
Naloxone
(Acronym: LEAN)

○ **If a drug is administered endotracheally what is the minimum recommended volume of fluid needed to overcome surface tension of the inside of the tube?**

3 - 5 ml of normal saline (if the drug volume to be administered ET is < 3-5 ml add saline until the total volume exceeds 3 ml).

○ **If a peripheral vein is utilized to administer a drug, it is recommended to flush the line with what volume of normal saline?**

5 ml of normal saline should be used to move the drug along.

O **The intraosseous route for drug administration is limited to children of what age group?**

6 years of age or younger.

O **When a medication is added to a solution for infusion, what must be done to the IV tubing in order to assure immediate delivery of the agent?**

The mixed solution must be run through the delivery system to the point where the IV tubing attaches to the hub of the IV catheter.

O **Many drugs used in resuscitation have specific effects on target organs. Epinephrine, Dopamine, Dobutamine and isoproterenol have either Alpha- or Beta-receptor activity or both. What does Alpha activity do?**

Alpha activity causes vasoconstriction.

O **What does Beta activity do?**

Beta activity causes the heart to beat faster and harder
Beta activity also causes vasodilatation and bronchodilation

O **What are the expected pharmacologic effects of epinephrine?**

Increased cardiac automaticity (Beta)
Increased heart rate (Beta)
Increased cardiac contractility (Beta)
Increased systemic vascular resistance (Alpha)
Increased perfusion (Alpha/Beta combination effects)

O **What are the indications for the administration of epinephrine?**

Cardiac arrest (Alpha)
Symptomatic bradycardia that will not respond to oxygenation and ventilation (Beta)
Hypotension not responding to volume resuscitation (Alpha/Beta combination)

O **What is the most important therapeutic effect from the administration of epinephrine during CPR?**

The Alpha effect. This effect enhances coronary and CNS perfusion during CPR.

O **What is the recommended initial IV or intraosseous dose of epinephrine for the management of symptomatic bradycardia not responding to oxygenation and ventilation?**

0.01mg/kg (0.1ml/kg of a 1:10,000 solution).

❍   **What is the recommended initial IV or intraosseous dose of epinephrine for the management of cardiac arrest?**

0.01mg/kg (0.1ml/kg of a 1:10,000 solution).

❍   **What is recommended for a subsequent dose of epinephrine in persistent pulseless cardiac arrest?**

0.1mg/kg (0.1ml/kg of a 1:1000 solution) IV or intraosseous. Notation that high dose epinephrine does not improve outcome.

❍   **How often should epinephrine be administered in a cardiac arrest resuscitation?**

Every 3 - 5 minutes.

❍   **What is the endotracheal dose of epinephrine?**

0.1mg/kg (0.1ml/kg of a 1:1000 solution).

❍   **With what should the endotracheal dose of epinephrine be diluted?**

3 - 5ml of normal saline only if the volume of drug to be delivered is <3 ml.

❍   **What happens if epinephrine is added to or given through a line with bicarbonate?**

The epinephrine will become inactivated.

❍   **What are two post epinephrine administration side effects?**

Hypertension
Tachycardia

❍   **What narcotic agent is recommended in kids?**

Fentanyl citrate (Sublimaze) 2-4 mcg/kg IV or IM.

❍   **What is the duration of action of Fentanyl?**

1-2 hours.

❍   **What is the advantage of Fentanyl over other opioids?**

Less histamine release and associated hypotension.

❍   **What is the generic name for Versed?**

Midazolam.

○   **What class of agent is Midazolam?**

A sedative hypnotic.

○   **What is the dosing regimen for Midazolam?**

0.1-0.2mg/kg (maximum 4mg) IV or IM, 1-2 hours.

○   **What is the most significant side effect of Midazolam?**

Respiratory depression.

○   **T/F: Midazolam has analgesic as well as sedative properties.**

False. That is why it is important to always give an analgesic in addition when performing painful procedures.

○   **What is the therapeutic effect of sodium bicarbonate (NaHCO₃)?**

Sodium bicarbonate buffers the blood and reverses metabolic acidosis.

○   **Why is it important to be able to adequately ventilate a patient who has received sodium bicarbonate?**

$NaHCO_3$ (Sodium Bicarbonate) generates an increase in CO_2 production as the hydrogen ion is buffered – adequate ventilation is necessary to remove the additional load to CO_2.

○   **When should sodium bicarbonate be considered for administration?**

When severe acidosis is associated with prolonged cardiac arrest, shock, hyperkalemia or tricyclic antidepressant toxicity.

○   **What is the initial dose for sodium bicarbonate when a base deficit cannot be determined?**

1 mEq/kg IV or intraosseous.

○   **What is the subsequent dose of sodium bicarbonate when a base deficit cannot be determined?**

0.5mEq/kg IV.

○   **How often may sodium bicarbonate be repeated?**

Every 10 minutes during prolonged cardiac arrest.

❍   **How fast should sodium bicarbonate be administered?**

Slowly over 1-2 minutes.

❍   **T/F: Excessive administration of sodium bicarbonate may result in metabolic alkalosis.**

True.

❍   **T/F: Administration of sodium bicarbonate can result in lowering serum potassium.**

True.

❍   **What is the standard adult concentration of sodium bicarbonate?**

8.4%.

❍   **What is the standard pediatric concentration of sodium bicarbonate?**

4.2%.

❍   **What should be done with the IV tubing before and after sodium bicarbonate has been given?**
The IV tubing should be flushed with normal saline.

❍   **Is atropine a sympathetic or a parasympathetic blocker?**

A parasympathetic blocker.

❍   **T/F: Parasympathetic stimulation is the same as vagal stimulation.**

True.

❍   **What effect does atropine have on the heart rate?**

Atropine will cause the heart rate to increase.

❍   **What are two cardiovascular conditions for which atropine administration is indicated?**

Asystolic cardiac arrest
Hemodynamically significant bradycardia

❍   **What is the benefit of atropine administration to a child during endotracheal intubation attempts?**

Atropine can prevent vagally mediated bradycardia.

○ **What is the indicated heart rate for administration of atropine to a young child with poor perfusion?**

Less than 60 beats per minute.

○ **What is the recommended dose of atropine?**

0.02mg/kg IV or intraosseous (IO).

○ **What is the minimum IV/IO single dose of atropine for a child?**

0.1mg.

○ **What is the maximum IV/IO single dose of atropine for a child?**

0.5mg.

○ **What is the maximum total dose of atropine for a child?**

1 mg.

○ **What is the maximum total dose of atropine for an adolescent?**

2 mg.

○ **How often may atropine be repeated?**

5 minutes after initial administration if symptoms persist.

○ **What may atropine administrated at lower than recommended doses do to the heart rate?**

Cause a paradoxical slowing of the heart rate.

○ **What is the recommended dose of atropine to be administered endotracheally?**

Two to three times the IV/IO dose.

○ **T/F: The pupillary dilatation associated with atropine will not react (constrict) to light reflex.**

False. The pupils will still constrict.

○ **Naloxone (Narcan) is indicated for what condition?**

Narcotic (opiate) toxicity induced symptoms.

❍   **What are three significant symptoms associated with narcotic (opiate) intoxication?**

Respiratory depression
CNS depression
Hypoperfusion

❍   **What is the onset of effect for naloxone (Narcan)?**

< 2 minutes.

❍   **What is the duration of activity for naloxone (Narcan)?**

Around 45 minutes.

❍   **By what routes may naloxone (Narcan) be administered?**

IV, IO and ETT.

❍   **What is the recommended IV/IO dose of naloxone (Narcan) for infants and children up to 20kg?**

0.1mg/kg.

❍   **Children weighing more than 20kg may be given IV/IO Narcan at what dose?**

2 mg.

❍   **What is the recommended infusion rate for Narcan?**

0.04 - 0.16mg/kg/hour.

❍   **What may occur after administration of naloxone (Narcan) if the narcotic effect is abruptly reversed?**

Acute narcotic withdrawal.

❍   **What are the symptoms of acute narcotic withdrawal?**

Nausea and vomiting, tachycardia, hypertension, seizures and cardiac dysrhythmias.

❍   **Why is hypoglycemia bad?**

Because it is important for cells to function normally especially in the brain. Hypoglycemia can precipitate seizure activity and depress myocardial function.

❍   **T/F: You can safely administer glucose without knowing the existing serum glucose concentrations.**

False. It is important to determine serum glucose concentration prior to the administration of glucose.

❍   **When should glucose administration be considered?**

When hypoglycemia is present or the infant or child fails to respond to standard resuscitation measures.

❍   **What is the dosage range of glucose?**

0.5 - 1.0gm/kg IV or IO.

❍   **What is the maximum recommended concentration of glucose for administration to children?**

25% (D25W).

❍   **When dextrose is supplied as 50% (D50W), what is the dilution to reduce the concentration to 25% (D25W)?**

1:1 with sterile water.

❍   **What is the dilution to reduce the concentration to 10% (D10W)?**

1:4 with sterile water.

❍   **What are three conditions that can lead to poor outcomes if high concentration glucose (D50/D25) is administered to children?**

Children with head injuries
Near drowning (submersion)
Shock

❍   **What effect does calcium have on the normal, healthy myocardium?**

Calcium increases myocardial contractile function.

❍   **What are four indications for administration of calcium?**

Documented or suspected hypocalcemia
Hyperkalemia
Hypermagnesemia
Calcium channel blocker overdose

❍ **Calcium chloride 10% is equal to how many milligrams per milliliter?**

100mg/ml.

❍ **What is the recommended dose of calcium chloride?**

20mg/kg IV.

❍ **How fast should calcium chloride be pushed?**

Not to exceed 100mg/min.

❍ **Why should you avoid mixing calcium chloride with sodium bicarbonate?**

Because it forms a precipitate.

❍ **What may happen if calcium is administered too fast?**

Bradycardia or asystole may occur.

❍ **Why should calcium only be administered through a large, well-secured intravenous line?**

Because calcium can cause significant chemical damage if it infiltrates into surrounding tissue.

❍ **What does prostaglandin E1 do?**

Prevents closure of the ductus arteriosis in newborns.

❍ **What are the indications for administration of prostaglandin E1?**

Infants with congenital cardiovascular disease with ductal dependent lesions

❍ **What are the signs and symptoms, in the newborn, associated with congenital cardiovascular abnormalities that could indicate the need for administration of prostaglandin E1?**

Cyanosis or shock.

❍ **How should prostaglandin E1 be administered?**

Continuous intravenous infusion.

❍ **Why should prostaglandin E1 be administered by continuous intravenous infusion?**

It has a very short half-life.

❍   **What is the effective dose range of prostaglandin E1?**

0.05 - 0.10 mcg/kg/min.

❍   **What are ten potential adverse reactions associated with the administration of prostaglandin E1?**

Apnea
Hypotension
Hyperpyrexia
Jitteriness
Diarrhea
Cardiac dysrhythmias
Hypocalcemia
Hypoglycemia
Renal Failure
Coagulopathies

❍   **Because prostaglandin E1 may cause apnea, what should you be prepared to do during its administration?**

Secure the airway with an endotracheal tube and oxygenate/ventilate the infant.

❍   **What are the indications for the administration of epinephrine via continuous IV infusion?**

Hemodynamically significant bradycardia
Asystolic or pulseless cardiac arrest
Prevailing poor perfusion not responding to volume replacement and in the presence of a
    stable cardiac rhythm

❍   **What is the infusion range for IV continuous infusion of epinephrine?**

0.01mcg/kg/min. - 1.0mcg/kg/min. titrated to desired response.

❍   **What is the recommended preparation formula for IV continuous epinephrine infusion?**

0.6 x patient weight (kg) = amount of epinephrine (mg) added to 100ml crystalloid.

❍   **When mixed appropriately, how may the epinephrine infusion rate be calculated?**

By setting the infusion rate to 1ml/hour the delivery of epinephrine will equal
0.1mcg/kg/min.

❍   **What are five potential adverse reactions associated with epinephrine infusion?**

Tachycardia
Ventricular dysrhythmias
Profound peripheral vasoconstriction
Compromised renal and hepatic blood flow
Local infiltration may cause ischemic tissue damage

❍ **What are the indications for the administration of dopamine?**

Hypotension and poor peripheral perfusion not responding to volume replacement and in the presence of a stable cardiac rhythm.

❍ **What is the dose range for IV dopamine infusion?**

2 - 20mcg/kg/min. titrated to desired response.

❍ **What is the recommended preparation formula for IV dopamine infusion?**

6mg x patient weight (kg) = amount of dopamine (mg) to be added to 100ml crystalloid.

❍ **When mixed appropriately, how may the dopamine infusion rate be calculated?**

By setting the infusion rate to 1ml/hour the delivery of dobutamine will equal 1mcg/kg/min.

❍ **What are five potential adverse reactions associated with dopamine administration?**

Tachycardia
Ventricular dysrhythmias
Profound peripheral vasoconstriction
Compromised renal and hepatic blood flow
Local infiltration may cause ischemic tissue damage

❍ **What are the two major indications for the administration of dobutamine infusion?**

Cardiogenic shock
Septic shock

❍ **What is the dose range for IV dobutamine infusion?**

2 - 20mcg/kg/min. titrated to the desired response.

❍ **What is the recommended preparation formula for IV dobutamine infusion?**

6mg x patient weight (kg) = amount of dobutamine (mg) to be added to 100ml crystalloid.

O   When mixed appropriately, how may the dobutamine infusion rate be calculated?

By setting the infusion rate to 1ml/hour the delivery of dobutamine will equal 1mcg/kg/min.

O   What are four potential adverse reactions associated with dobutamine administration?

Tachycardia
Ventricular dysrhythmias
Hypertension or hypotension
Local infiltration may cause ischemic tissue damage

O   What are three indications for the administration of lidocaine by IV bolus?

Ventricular dysrhythmias
Ventricular tachycardia
Ventricular fibrillation (after defibrillation)

O   What is the recommended dose of lidocaine IV bolus?

1mg/kg (not to exceed 3mg/kg).

O   What are the indications for the infusion of lidocaine?

Ventricular dysrhythmias
Ventricular tachycardia
Ventricular fibrillation (after defibrillation)

O   When should lidocaine infusion be started?

Following effective lidocaine bolus administration.

O   What is the recommended dose range of lidocaine infusion?

20-50mcg/kg/min. titrated to desired response.

O   What is the recommended preparation formula for IV lidocaine infusion?

Mix 120mg lidocaine in 100ml crystalloid.

O   When mixed appropriately, how may the lidocaine infusion rate be calculated?

By setting the infusion rate to:
   1ml/hour the delivery of lidocaine will equal 20mcg/kg/min

2.5ml/hr the delivery of lidocaine will equal 50mcg/kg/min

❍   **What are three potential adverse reactions associated with lidocaine administration?**

Myocardial depression
Hypotension
Central nervous system manifestations, such as drowsiness, disorientation, muscle
    twitching and seizures

❍   **What are the indications for the administration of adenosine?**

Supraventricular tachycardia (heart rates >220 BPM) with or without evidence of poor
perfusion.

❍   **What is the recommended dose of adenosine?**

0.1 - 0.2mg/kg IV rapid bolus.

❍   **What are the indications for the use of Amiodarone in children?**

Wide range of atrial and ventricular arrhythmias, particularly ectopic atrial tachycardia,
junctional ectopic tachycardia, and ventricular tachycardia.

❍   **What are the two main precautions when using Amiodarone?**

May produce hypotension
May prolong QT interval and increase propensity for polymorphic ventricular
    arrhythmias

❍   **With what antiarrhythmic should you avoid using Amiodarone?**

Procainamide.

❍   **What is the half-life of Amiodarone?**

Up to 40 days!

❍   **What is the dosing of Amiodarone in refractory pulseless VT, VF?**

5mg/kg rapid IV/IO bolus.

❍   **What is the dosing of Amiodarone for perfusing supraventricular and ventricular arrhythmias?**

Loading dose: 5mg/kg IV/IO over 20 to 60 minutes (repeat to a maximum of 15mg/kg
per day IV).

CARDIAC RHYTHM DISTURBANCES

"Times are bad. Children no longer obey their parents, and everyone is writing a book."
~ Cicero ~

"In infants and children, life-threatening cardiac rhythm disturbances are more frequently the result rather than the cause of acute cardiovascular emergencies. Primary cardiac arrest is uncommon in this age group. Typically, cardiac arrest is the end result of hypoxemia and acidosis resulting from respiratory insufficiency or shock. Thus, in the pediatric age group attention must first be directed toward establishment of a patent airway, effective ventilation, adequate oxygenation, and circulatory stabilization. This chapter is limited to a discussion of the arrhythmias most commonly associated with emergency situations requiring CPR and is not intended to be a comprehensive review of pediatric cardiac arrhythmias."

❍ **T/F: In infants and children, life-threatening cardiac rhythm disturbances are more frequently the cause rather than the result of cardiovascular emergencies.**

False. In infants and children, life-threatening cardiac rhythm disturbances are more frequently the result rather than the cause of cardiovascular emergencies.

❍ **Which is more common in infants and children, primary or secondary cardiac arrest?**

Secondary.

❍ **Typically, what is cardiac arrest the result of in children?**

It is the end result of hypoxemia and acidosis resulting from respiratory insufficiency or shock.

❍ **Toward what four things must attention first be directed when confronted with life-threatening cardiac arrhythmias in children?**

Toward establishment of a patent airway, effective ventilation, adequate oxygenation, and circulatory stabilization.

❍ **Define the surface electrocardiogram.**

The surface electrocardiogram is a graphic representation of the electrical sequence of myocardial depolarization and repolarization.

○   **What three waveforms does a normal cardiac cycle consist of?**

P, QRS, and T wave.

○   **Where does electrical depolarization begin in the myocardium?**

Electrical depolarization begins in the sinoatrial node.

○   **Where is the sinoatrial node located?**

At the junction of the superior vena cava and the right atrium.

○   **After leaving the sinoatrial node, what is the pathway of electrical depolarization?**

It advances via atrial tissue and the internodal pathways to the atrioventricular junctional tissue.

○   **What happens to depolarization at the atrioventricular junction?**

It slows temporarily.

○   **Where does it go then?**

It then progresses via the bundle of His and its divisions to depolarize the ventricular myocardium.

○   **What is the first deflection on the surface ECG called?**

The P wave.

○   **What does the P wave signify?**

It represents the depolarization of both atria.

○   **What does the PR interval represent?**

The delay in conduction at the AV junction and the time to spread the impulse through the bundle of His.

○   **What represents the depolarization of the ventricles?**

The QRS complex.

○   **What do the ST segment and the T wave represent?**

Ventricular repolarization.

○ **What are the two key factors in influencing differences in normal heart rate in children?**

Age and physical activity.

○ **What two primary pathological conditions may influence heart rate in children?**

Fever and volume loss (fluid loss, e.g. vomiting or diarrhea, and hemorrhage).

○ **T/F: A febrile infant with normal cardiovascular function can have a heart rate of 200 beats per minute or higher.**

True. These infants can have heart rates up to 200 + beats per minute, heart rates in infants and young children ≥ 220 often are caused a tachyarrhythmia (supraventricular tachycardia).

○ **When should you continuously monitor the ECG in children?**

When they have evidence of respiratory or cardiovascular instability, including children who have sustained a cardiopulmonary arrest.

○ **What can the ECG tell you about the effectiveness of myocardial contractility and the quality of tissue perfusion?**

Nothing.

○ **With what must you correlate information derived from the ECG in the treatment of children?**

Clinical evaluation.

○ **What interval is measured on the ECG to determine heart rate?**

The R-R interval.

○ **T/F: Never use adult ECG patches on children.**

False. Adult patches may be used by trimming excess tape from the electrodes to make them smaller.

○ **Where are metal electrodes usually attached?**

To the extremities.

○ **Why should electrodes be placed at the periphery of the anterior chest?**

To avoid interference with chest compressions if CPR becomes necessary.

○ **Why is it advantageous to avoid placing electrodes on the anterior chest?**

So they won't interfere with auscultation of the heart and lungs, and chest radiographs will be free of radiopaque artifact.

○ **What is the typical electrode placement on children?**

The shoulders or the lateral chest surfaces, and the ground electrode are usually placed on the abdomen or thigh.

○ **What is the most common cause of asystole on ECG?**

A loose electrode or wire.

○ **What are the four most common artifacts commonly observed on ECG?**

A straight line due to a loose lead
A tall T wave counted as an R wave by the tachometer
Absence of P waves due to lead placement
60-cycle interference

○ **When should a rhythm disturbance in a child be treated as an emergency?**

Only if it compromises cardiac output or has the potential to degenerate into a lethal (collapse) rhythm.

○ **What is the equation for determining cardiac output?**

Stroke volume times heart rate.

○ **Why can cardiac output diminish as a result of very rapid rates?**

Because they may compromise diastolic filling and therefore stroke volume.

○ **In the setting of acute emergencies, cardiac rhythm disturbances should be classified according to their effect on central pulses. These three classifications are:**

Fast pulse rate = tachyarrhythmia
Slow pulse rate = bradyarrhythmia
Absent pulse = pulseless arrest (collapse rhythm)

○ **What are the two primary cardiac rhythms that result in excessively fast rates?**

Supraventricular and ventricular tachycardias.

❍ **What is the most rapid and effective method of treating tachyarrhythmias that result in cardiovascular instability and signs of shock?**

Synchronized cardioversion.

❍ **What is the cause of slow rhythms associated with cardiovascular instability in infants and children?**

AV block or suppression of normal sinus node impulse generation caused by hypoxemia or acidosis.

❍ **What does the initial therapy for these slow rhythms consist of?**

Establishment of a patent airway, provision of adequate ventilation and oxygenation, and administration of medications to improve perfusion (i.e., sympathomimetics).

❍ **With what dysrhythmias is the absence of palpable pulses associated?**

Asystole, ventricular fibrillation, pulseless ventricular tachycardia, or a pulseless electrical activity, such as electromechanical dissociation.

❍ **Define sinus tachycardia in children.**

A rate of sinus node discharge higher than normal for age.

❍ **What is the typical physiological cause of sinus tachycardia?**

The need for increased cardiac output or oxygen delivery.

❍ **Is sinus tachycardia a true arrhythmia?**

No, it is often a nonspecific clinical sign rather than a true arrhythmia.

❍ **Name six common causes of sinus tachycardia.**

Anxiety, fever, pain, blood loss, sepsis, shock.

❍ **What is the normal awake heart rate in infants newborn to three months?**

85-205.

❍ **Is sinus tachycardia regular or irregular?**

Regular, but far less regular than SVT.

❍ **Describe P wave morphology in sinus tachycardia.**

Normal, upright.

O   **What is the wave sequence in sinus tachycardia?**

Regular P-QRS-T sequence.

O   **Describe QRS duration in sinus tachycardia.**

Normal.

O   **What is the therapy for sinus tachycardia?**

Therapy is directed at treating the underlying cause.

O   **Why are attempts to decrease the heart rate by pharmacological means inappropriate in sinus tachycardia?**

Because it is a symptom, not a cause.

O   **Is supraventricular tachycardia (SVT) a regular or irregular rhythm?**

Regular.

O   **T/F: SVT is often paroxysmal.**

True.

O   **What is the most common cause of SVT?**

A reentry mechanism that involves an accessory pathway and/or the AV conduction system.

O   **Which patient is least likely to tolerate SVT well: small infants, infants, or older children?**

Although SVT is usually well tolerated in most infants and older children, it can lead to cardiovascular collapse and clinical evidence of shock in some small infants.

O   **What is the usual heart rate of infants in SVT?**

Greater than or equal to 220 bpm but often higher.

O   **What is the usual P wave morphology in SVT?**

P waves may not be visible, especially when the ventricular rate is high.

O   **What is the QRS duration in SVT?**

QRS duration is often normal (less than 0.08 seconds) in most (>90%) children.

○ **With what rhythm is SVT with aberrant conduction usually confused?**

Ventricular tachycardia, but this form of SVT is rare in infants and children.

○ **What ST and T wave changes may be observed in SVT?**

ST and T wave changes consistent with myocardial ischemia may be observed if tachycardia persists.

○ **With what rhythm is narrow complex SVT in children easily confused?**

Extreme sinus tachycardia associated with sepsis or hypovolemia, particularly because either rhythm may be associated with poor systemic perfusion.

○ **What three things may help you distinguish SVT from sinus tachycardia?**

Heart rate, ECG, variability.

○ **How can heart rate help you distinguish SVT from sinus tachycardia?**

Sinus tachycardia is usually associated with a heart rate less than 200 bpm. In most (60%) infants with SVT, the heart rate is greater than 230 bpm.

○ **How can the ECG help you distinguish SVT from sinus tachycardia?**

P waves may be difficult to identify in both sinus tachycardia and SVT once the ventricular rate exceeds 200 bpm. If the P waves can be identified, the P wave axis is usually abnormal in SVT but normal in sinus tachycardia.

○ **How can variability help you distinguish SVT from sinus tachycardia?**

In sinus tachycardia, the rate may vary from beat to beat, but there is no beat-to-beat variation in SVT. Termination of SVT is abrupt, whereas the heat rate slows gradually in sinus tachycardia.

○ **In sum, what six indications would lead you to suspect sinus tachycardia?**

History compatible (fever, volume loss, hemorrhage or pain)
P waves present/normal
HR often varies with activity
Variable RR with constant PR
Infants: rate usually <220 bpm
Children: rate usually <180 bpm

○ **In sum, what six factors would lead you to suspect this was supraventricular**

tachycardia?

History incompatible (vague or nonspecific history or history of congenital heart disease)
P waves absent/abnormal
HR not variable with activity
Abrupt rate changes
Infants: rate usually >220 bpm
Children: rate usually >180 bpm

○   **What are the first three things you should do when you encounter a child with a rapid heart rate with evidence of poor perfusion?**

Assess and maintain the airway
Administer 100% oxygen
Ensure effective ventilation

○   **If the QRS duration is wide for the child's age, what dysrhythmia should you treat?**

Treat as presumptive ventricular tachycardia.

○   **Name two reversible causes of ventricular tachycardia in children.**

Electrolyte imbalance, drug toxicity.

○   **When should vagal maneuvers be attempted in children?**

In cases of stable SVT with a pulse. Should not delay adenosine therapy or cardioversion if poor perfusion is present.

○   **When should a 12-lead EKG be done?**

As soon as possible during treatment.

○   **What is the only difference between the Algorithm for Pediatric Tachycardia with Poor Perfusion and with Adequate Perfusion?**

With poor perfusion and no ability to get rapid IV placement cardioversion comes first. With adequate perfusion drugs come first.

○   **If rapid vascular access is available, what is your first line of treatment in symptomatic wide complex tachycardia in children?**

Amiodarone 5mg/kg IV over 20-60 minutes, or Procainamide 15mg/kg IV over 30-60 minutes, or Lidocaine 1mg/kg IV bolus (no cardioversion delays).

○   **T/F: Amiodarone and Procainamide should always be given together.**

False, do not routinely administer them together.

○   **If the antiarrhythmic doesn't work, what do you do next?**

Synchronized cardioversion.

○   **Under what circumstance should you delay synchronized cardioversion in the symptomatic child with wide complex tachycardia?**

Never delay cardioversion.

○   **What is the dosage for synchronized cardioversion?**

0.5-1 Joules/kg. Repeat cardioversion as needed.

○   **If conversion with lidocaine was successful, at what rate should you start a lidocaine infusion?**

20-50 mcg/kg/minute.

○   **A two-month-old is brought into your ER by her mother, pale and with a CRT of > 2 seconds. Mom says she hasn't been acting right all day. Her heart rate is too fast to count. Monitor shows a probable SVT at 260 bpm. No IV access is available. What do you do?**

Synchronized cardioversion 0.5-1 J/kg.

○   **You have the same patient, but with a patent IV. What do you do?**

Adenosine 0.1 mg/kg followed by rapid NS bolus 2-5ml.

○   **What is unique about the way you administer adenosine?**

Proximal port
Both medication and flush syringe in same port
Very rapid sequential push
Keep your thumb on both syringes while pushing

○   **What do you do if the adenosine doesn't work?**

You may double the dose and repeat once.

○   **What is the maximum dose of adenosine?**

12 mg.

○   **What should you do if adenosine fails to convert the rhythm?**

If patient unstable, cardiovert.
If stable:
  12-lead ECG
  Reevaluate rhythm
  Consider sedation (no delays)
  Consider cardioversion for SVT
  Consider treatment for ST
  Consult pediatric cardiologist

○   **What four factors would cause you to lean toward a diagnosis of probable sinus tachycardia rather than SVT?**

P waves present and normal
Variable RR with constant PR
Infants: rate usually <220 bpm
Children: rate usually <180 bpm

○   **Name nine possible causes of sinus tachycardia.**

Fever
Shock
Pain
Hypovolemia
Hypoxia
Abnormal electrolytes
Drug ingestions
Pneumothorax
Cardiac tamponade

○   **What four factors would cause you to lean toward a diagnosis of probable supraventricular tachycardia over sinus tachycardia?**

P waves absent or abnormal
Abrupt rate change to or from normal
Infants: rate usually >220 bpm
Children: rate usually >180 bpm

○   **A seven-year-old boy is brought by his father to your clinic. His father says that he complained of a fluttering in his chest, but otherwise feels fine. He is alert and oriented, skin is warm and dry, CRT is < 2 seconds. His pulse is strong but too rapid to count. What do you do?**

Obtain a 12-lead ECG and evaluate QRS duration.

○   **You obtain a 12-lead ECG and the rate is 240 bpm. What is the normal QRS duration?**

Approximately ≤ 0.08 seconds.

○   **The QRS is 0.05 seconds. What do you need to determine in order to treat this patient?**

Whether the rhythm is ST or SVT.

○   **In analyzing the ECG, you notice that P waves are absent, and the rate is sustained at 240 bpm. What rhythm is this?**

Probable SVT.

○   **The patient remains stable. What should you do?**

Establish vascular access and give adenosine.

○   **You administer 0.1 mg/kg adenosine rapid IV push. There is no change in rhythm. What now?**

Double the dose.

○   **You double the dose and still no change. The patient remains stable. What now?**

Call the cardiologist. Monitor the patient for deterioration or rhythm change.

(NOTE: this is not a reasonable scenario – just create a new one)

○   **A 12 month-old male with history of congenital heart disease is brought to the ED by his mother for irritability. The boy is awake and you place the child on a monitor. A rate of 200 bpm is noted and the QRS complex is .15 seconds. How will the treatment for this patient be different than the previous patient?**

Do not administer adenosine. Because of the wide QRS complex treat as if it is ventricular in origin. First, identify and treat reversible causes, such as electrolyte imbalance and drug toxicity. Then, administer Amiodarone 5 mg/kg IV over 20 to 60 minutes **or** Procainamide 15 mg/kg IV over 30-60 minutes **or** Lidocaine 1mg/kg IV. May repeat Lidocaine twice as needed.

○   **Five minutes after you administer lidocaine, the rate suddenly drops to 88 and regular. The patient states the fluttering in his chest is gone. What now?**

Start a lidocaine infusion at 20-50 mcg/kg per minute. Keep waiting for the pediatric cardiologist.

○   **What is the treatment of choice for patients with tachyarrhythmias (SVT, VT, atrial fibrillation, atrial flutter) who show evidence of cardiovascular compromise?**

Synchronized cardioversion.

❍ **Why is synchronized cardioversion preferable to unsynchronized countershock?**

Synchronization of delivered energy with the ECG reduces the possibility of inducing VF, which can occur if an electrical impulse is delivered during the relative refractory period of the ventricle.

❍ **What is the initial energy dose for synchronized cardioversion?**

0.5 J/kg.

❍ **What is the second energy dose for synchronized cardioversion?**

1 J/kg.

❍ **If conversion to sinus rhythm does not occur after two doses of electricity, what should you reconsider?**

The diagnosis of SVT. ST may actually be present.

❍ **T/F: Ideally, infants and children should be ventilated with 100% oxygen before cardioversion.**

True.

❍ **T/F: Secure vascular access should be achieved prior to cardioversion.**

True.

❍ **What else should you consider before cardioversion?**

Vascular access and the administration of a sedative and analgesia. However, if shock is present, cardioversion should not be delayed while these therapies are instituted.

❍ **What is adenosine?**

An endogenous purine nucleoside that slows conduction through the AV node.

❍ **What does adenosine cause?**

It causes transient sinus bradycardia, and usually terminates SVT rapidly, safely and effectively.

❍ **What is the half-life of adenosine?**

Less than ten seconds.

○ **What is the duration of effect of adenosine?**

Less than two minutes.

○ **Why does adenosine have such a short half-life?**

It is rapidly sequestered by red blood cells.

○ **What are the primary indications for adenosine?**

It is the initial drug of choice for the diagnosis and treatment of SVT in infants and children.

○ **Why is adenosine so effective in terminating SVT in infants and children?**

Because SVT usually involves a reentrant pathway including the AV node in these patients.

○ **When may adenosine be ineffective in terminating SVT?**

If the arrhythmia is not due to a reentry rhythm involving the AV node or sinus node, e.g., atrial flutter, atrial fibrillation, or atrial or ventricular tachycardia.

○ **How may adenosine be of use in arrhythmias not involving reentry at the AV or sinus nodes?**

It will not terminate the arrhythmia but may produce a transient block at the AV node that may allow the health care provider to review the 12-lead ECG and determine the underlying rhythm.

○ **What is the recommended initial dose of adenosine?**

Rapid IV bolus of 0.1mg/kg followed immediately by a rapid bolus of at least 2 ml of normal saline.

○ **Why should you immediately push normal saline following adenosine?**

To push it quickly to the heart before the red blood cells have a chance to sequester it.

○ **What special technique should you use when administering adenosine?**

Draw up the medication and the flush and insert both needles into a proximal IV port. Clamp the IV line just above the injection port. Push the drug as rapidly as possible followed by the flush as rapidly as possible.

○ **Why is it important to use two hands to administer adenosine?**

One hand on the medication syringe, one on the flush. Maintain pressure on the plunger after pushing the drug to avoid having the flush pressure push the medication back into the medication syringe.

○   **If the initial dose of adenosine is ineffective, what should you do?**

Double it.

○   **What is the maximum dose of adenosine?**

The maximum single dose should usually not exceed 12 mg or 0.3 mg/kg.

○   **T/F: Adenosine may not be administered intraosseously.**

False. It may be administered intraosseously if other IV access is not available.

○   **What are the common side effects of adenosine?**

Flushing, dyspnea, chest pain, bradycardia, and irritability.

○   **How quickly do these side effects usually resolve?**

Within 1 to 2 minutes.

○   **With what group of patients should adenosine be used with caution?**

In children with denervated, transplanted hearts.
Adenosine is contraindicated in patients taking dipyridamole (Persantine) or carbamazepine (Tegretol) because these medications can further prolong the AV block caused by the administration of adenosine.

○   **What medications can block the receptor responsible for adenosine's electrophysiological effects?**

Therapeutic concentrations of theophylline or related methylxanthines (caffeine and theobromine).

○   **Can you still use adenosine in a child on theophylline?**

Yes, but he or she may require a larger dose than usual.

○   **What is verapamil?**

A calcium channel blocker.

○   **How does verapamil exert its antiarrhythmic effect?**

By slowing conduction and prolonging the effective refractory period in the AV junctional tissue.

○ **What effect of verapamil may cause myocardial depression?**

Its negative inotropic effect.

○ **What negative consequences have been observed with verapamil?**

Profound bradycardia, hypotension, and asystole.

○ **In what patients should verapamil not be used?**

It should not be used to treat SVT in an emergency setting in infants less than 1 year of age, in children with congestive heart failure or myocardial depression, in children receiving beta-adrenergic-blocking drugs, or in those who may have a bypass tract.

○ **T/F: Ventricular tachycardia (VT) is common in the pediatric age group.**

False. It is uncommon.

○ **What is the ventricular rate range of VT?**

The ventricular rate may vary from 120 to 400 beats per minute.

○ **T/F: VT with a slow ventricular rate can be well tolerated.**

True.

○ **Why is rapid VT not well tolerated?**

It compromises stroke volume and cardiac output and may degenerate into ventricular fibrillation.

○ **Which children are most likely to develop VT?**

Those with underlying structural heart disease or prolonged QT syndrome.

○ **What are some of the non-congenital causes of VT?**

Acute hypoxemia, hypothermia, acidosis, electrolyte imbalance, drug toxicity (e.g., tricyclic antidepressants, digoxin toxicity), and poisons.

○ **Describe the ventricular rate for VT.**

At least 120 beats per minute and regular.

○ **Describe the QRS in VT.**

The QRS is wide (greater than 0.08 seconds).

❍ **Describe the P waves in VT.**

P waves are not identifiable. When present, they will not be related to the QRS (AV dissociation). At slower rates the atria may be depolarized in a retrograde manner, and therefore there will be a 1:1 VA association.

❍ **Describe the T waves in VT.**

T waves are usually opposite in polarity to the QRS.

❍ **What other dysrhythmia can look like VT?**

SVT with aberrant conduction. Fortunately, aberrant conduction is present in less than 10% of children with SVT.

❍ **T/F: Previously undiagnosed wide QRS tachycardia in an infant or child should be treated as VT until proven otherwise.**

True.

❍ **How should you treat VT without palpable pulses?**

Like ventricular fibrillation (VF).

❍ **If VT is associated with signs of shock (low cardiac output, poor perfusion), but pulses are palpable, what is the indicated treatment?**

Synchronized cardioversion.

❍ **What should be done if possible prior to cardioversion?**

Intubate and ventilate with 100% oxygen, secure vascular access, provide adequate sedation and analgesia.

❍ **Why is lidocaine useful in defibrillation?**

It raises the threshold for VF.

❍ **Why should lidocaine be given prior to cardioversion?**

It suppresses postcardioversion ventricular ectopy.

❍ **What is the dose of lidocaine given prior to cardioversion?**

A loading dose of 1 mg/kg followed by an infusion at 20-50 mcg/kg/minute.

○ **When is it inappropriate to give lidocaine prior to cardioversion?**

In an unstable child if the drug is not readily available or if vascular access has not been achieved.

○ **When should a lidocaine drip be considered following the return of spontaneous circulation after VT or VF?**

If the ventricular arrhythmias are thought to be associated with myocarditis or structural heart disease.

○ **How would you prepare a lidocaine infusion?**

Add 120mg lidocaine to 100ml 5% dextrose in water.

○ **What is the resulting concentration?**

1.2mg/ml.

○ **What is the infusion rate?**

1-2.5ml/kg/minute.

○ **What is an alternative method of mixing the infusion?**

Multiply 60 by the kilogram body weight to determine the amount of lidocaine (in milligrams) to be added to a solution of 5% dextrose in water for a total volume of 100 ml. Infusion of 2-5ml per hour of this solution will provide 20-50mcg/kg/minute.

○ **To ensure adequate plasma concentration, what should you do prior to starting the infusion?**

Administer a bolus of 1mg/kg.

○ **What effects can excessive plasma concentrations of lidocaine have?**

Myocardial and circulatory depression and possible central nervous system symptoms, including drowsiness, disorientation, muscle twitching, or seizures.

○ **When should you consider a reduced lidocaine infusion?**

If reduced lidocaine clearance is suspected, such as might occur in patients with shock or chronic congestive heart failure.

○ **In patients where reduced lidocaine clearance is suspected, what should be the infusion dose?**

A maximum of 20 mcg/kg/minute.

○ **T/F: There are no data on the usefulness of bretylium tosylate in the pediatric age group.**

True. (Besides, Bretylium is no longer commercially available.)

○ **What are the most common terminal rhythms in children?**

Sinus bradycardia, sinus node arrest with a slow junctional or ventricular escape rhythm, and various degrees of AV block.

○ **What are the most common causes of bradycardic rhythms?**

Hypoxemia, hypotension, and acidosis.

○ **Describe the P waves in bradycardia.**

P waves may or may not be visible.

○ **What is QRS duration in bradycardia?**

QRS duration may be normal or prolonged depending on the pacemaker focus.

○ **What is the relationship between P waves and the QRS complexes?**

The P and QRS may be unrelated (AV dissociation).

○ **If blood pressure is normal, should you treat bradycardia?**

If there is poor systemic perfusion, it should be treated regardless of blood pressure.

○ **What is the treatment for bradycardia?**

Adequate ventilation with 100% oxygen must be ensured, chest compressions performed, and epinephrine and atropine are administered as necessary.

○ **What is epinephrine?**

Epinephrine is a catecholamine with both alpha and beta-adrenergic receptor-stimulating action.

○ **What does beta-adrenergic action do?**

Increases myocardial contractility and heart rate.

○ **What is the recommended initial intravenous or intraosseous dose of epinephrine for the treatment of symptomatic bradycardia unresponsive to**

ventilation and oxygen administration?

0.01 mg/kg of the 1:10,000 solution (0.1 ml/kg).

○ **What is the dose given via the endotracheal tube?**

0.1 mg/kg of the 1:1,000 solution (0.1 ml/kg), diluted to a volume of 3-5 ml prior to instillation.

○ **What is atropine sulphate?**

A parasympathetic drug that accelerates sinus or atrial pacemakers and enhances AV conduction.

○ **When should atropine be used to treat bradycardia in infants and children?**

Only after adequate ventilation and oxygenation have been ensured, since hypoxemia is a common cause of bradycardia. Atropine may be used to treat vagally mediated bradycardia or primary AV block. Atropine may also be used to treat the effect of vagal stimulation during intubation. Epinephrine should be used to treat bradycardia associated with clinical evidence of shock.

○ **Why must a minimum dose of atropine be administered?**

Smaller doses may produce paradoxical bradycardia.

○ **What is the recommended dose of atropine?**

0.02 mg/kg, with a minimum dose of 0.1 mg and a maximum dose of 0.5 mg for a child and 1 mg for an adolescent.

○ **How often may the dose of atropine be repeated?**

Every five minutes to a maximum total dose of 1 mg for a child and 2 mg for an adolescent.

○ **What is the endotracheal dose of atropine?**

Absorption into the circulation by this route may be unreliable. The intravenous dose should be increased by two to three times and diluted to a minimum volume of 3-5 ml for endotracheal instillation.

○ **What do I do if I administer atropine and a tachycardia results?**

Tachycardia that follows atropine administration is usually sinus tachycardia and is usually well tolerated in the pediatric patient.

○ **What are the three cardiac mechanisms of pulseless arrest?**

Asystole, ventricular fibrillation, or a form of pulseless electrical activity (including electromechanical dissociation).

○ **What is asystole?**

Asystole is a form of pulseless arrest associated with absent cardiac electrical activity.

○ **Why is it essential to confirm asystole clinically?**

Clinical confirmation (absent pulse, absent spontaneous respirations, poor perfusion) is mandatory since a straight line can also be caused by a loose ECG monitoring lead.

○ **How does asystole appear on the monitor?**

Straight line. P waves are occasionally observed.

○ **What should be done immediately on determining pulselessness in asystole?**

Begin CPR; confirm cardiac rhythm in more than one lead.

○ **After beginning CPR, what should be done next?**

Secure airway, ventilate with 100% oxygen, and obtain IV or IO access.

○ **Your team is performing CPR on a pulseless and apneic 3 year old. The patient has been intubated, and IO access confirmed. What is the next step?**

Epinephrine IO 0.01 or 0.1 mg/kg repeated every 3-5 minutes.

○ **In the same scenario above, you show a sinus rhythm on the monitor. What is this called?**

Pulseless electrical activity (PEA).

○ **What is the most important thing to do, after initiating CPR, in treating PEA?**

Determine the cause. Without determining and treating the cause, the outlook is grim indeed.

○ **What are the six possible causes of pediatric bradycardia identified by PALS?**

Hypoxemia
Hypothermia
Head injury
Heart block

Heart transplant
Toxins/poisons/drugs

O   **What are some of the other causes you can think of?**

Spinal shock
Sepsis
Toxicity/overdose
Electrolyte imbalance
Myocarditis
Congenital cardiac anomaly

O   **If the bradycardia is not causing severe cardiopulmonary compromise, what should you do?**

Observe, support ABCs, consider transfer or transport to an ALS facility.

O   **If bradycardia is causing severe symptoms despite oxygenation and ventilation, what should you do?**

Perform chest compressions and administer epinephrine (IV/IO 0.01 mg/kg = 1/10,000 0.1 ml/kg, ET 0.1 mg/kg = 0.1 ml/kg 1/1,000.

O   **If perfusion continues to be poor after epinephrine, what should you do?**

Administer atropine 0.02 mg/kg (minimum dose 0.1 mg).

O   **How many doses of atropine can you give?**

2.

O   **When should you give atropine before epinephrine?**

For bradycardia due to suspected increase in vagal tone or primary AV block.

O   **If serious signs and symptoms continue after epinephrine and atropine, what should you do?**

Consider cardiac pacing.

O   **Refractory symptomatic bradycardia is most likely to degenerate into what rhythm?**

Pulseless electrical activity (PEA).

O   **The Pediatric Pulseless Arrest Algorithm divides pulseless arrest into two major categories. What are they?**

VF/VT
Not VF/VT (includes PEA and Asystole)

O   **What is ventricular fibrillation (VF)?**

A chaotic, disorganized series of depolarizations that result in quivering myocardium without organized contraction. This uncoordinated contraction of the ventricle does not result in significant cardiac output, so pulses are not palpable.

O   **Is VF a common terminal event in the pediatric age group?**

No, it is documented in only about 10% of children in whom a terminal rhythm is recorded.

O   **Is resuscitation outcome better if VF or asystole/PEA is the underlying rhythm on initial presentation in the pediatric age group?**

Resuscitation outcome is considerably better in VF.

O   **What is the initial therapy when an infant or child is pulseless?**

Establishment of adequate ventilation and oxygenation and provision of manual external chest compressions.

O   **When should defibrillation be attempted?**

Only if VF is confirmed by ECG monitoring.

O   **How is pulseless ventricular tachycardia (VT) treated?**

In the same manner as VF.

O   **What is the morphology of P, QRS, and T waves in VF?**

There are no identifiable P, QRS and T waves.

O   **How can VF waves be classified?**

VF waves are chaotic and can be classified as course or fine by the height of the waves (however, treatment is identical for all classifications of VF).

O   **What is the definitive treatment for VF or pulseless VT?**

Prompt defibrillation. However, ventilation with 100% oxygen and chest compressions should be continued until the moment of defibrillation. Ideally, vascular access is secured, but defibrillation should not be delayed to achieve this access.

❍ **T/F: Defibrillation should be attempted in asystole.**

False. Unless there is reasonable doubt that the dysrhythmia may actually be VF.

❍ **What is defibrillation?**

The untimed (asynchronous) depolarization of a critical mass of myocardial cells to allow spontaneous organized myocardial depolarization to resume.

❍ **What will happen if organized depolarization does not resume after defibrillation?**

VF will continue or will progress to electrical silence, at which point restoration of spontaneous cardiac activity may be impossible.

❍ **How does synchronized cardioversion differ from defibrillation?**

Synchronized cardioversion also results in depolarization of the myocardium, but cardioversion provides depolarization that is timed (synchronous) with the patient's intrinsic electrical activity.

❍ **Why is synchronized cardioversion inappropriate in the patient with VF?**

VF has no organized cardiac electrical activity with which to synchronize.

❍ **Successful defibrillation requires the passage of sufficient electric current (amperes) through the heart. On what two factors does this current flow depend?**

The energy (joules) provided and the transthoracic impedance (ohms), which is the resistance to current flow.

❍ **If transthoracic impedance is high, what must be done to achieve sufficient current for successful defibrillation or cardioversion?**

Increase the electrical current.

❍ **What eight factors determine transthoracic impedance?**

Energy selected
Electrode size
Paddle-skin coupling material
Number of shocks
Time intervals between shocks
Phase of ventilation
Size of chest
Paddle electrode pressure

○   **What is the optimal energy dose for defibrillation in infants and children?**

Trick question: the optimal energy dose has not been established (sorry).

○   **Although available information does not demonstrate a relation between energy dose and weight, pediatricians are committed to that relationship, with or without evidence! So what starting dose has been arbitrarily recommended for defibrillation?**

2 joules/kg, until further notice (or data is available).

○   **What can the operator do to minimize transthoracic impedance?**

Apply firm pressure to the paddles. Use an appropriate conduction medium.

○   **What should you do if the initial dose doesn't work?**

Double it.

○   **Why should you deliver the second dose as soon as possible after the first?**

Because the first dose reduces transthoracic impedance. And VF isn't too good for the kid.

○   **If the second shock doesn't work, what should you do?**

Give a third at the same energy level as the second.

○   **How long should you delay between the first three shocks?**

Just long enough to charge the paddles and check the rhythm with the paddles in place.

○   **Should you pause for CPR between shocks?**

No, unless there will be a delay due to equipment malfunction or other calamity.

○   **If VF continues after three shocks, what should you do?**

Administer epinephrine.

○   **After administration of epinephrine, how many times should you shock?**

The AHA 2000 guidelines give you a choice. Either once or three times.

○   **T/F: If VF continues despite the three defibrillation attempts, energy levels may need to be increased further.**

True, but ventilation with 100% oxygen, chest compressions and epinephrine should precede further defibrillation attempts.

○   **After CPR, defibrillation, and epinephrine, what medications should you consider?**

Amiodarone, Lidocaine, or Magnesium.

○   **What is it important to remember to do after administering each drug?**

Circulate with good CPR for 30-60 seconds before shocking.

○   **What is the initial dose of amiodarone in pediatric cardiac arrest?**

5mg/kg bolus IV/IO.

○   **What is the initial dose of lidocaine in pediatric cardiac arrest?**

1mg/kg bolus IV/IO/ET.

○   **When should magnesium be given in pediatric cardiac arrest?**

Torsades de pointes or hypomagnesemia.

○   **What is the initial dose of magnesium in pediatric cardiac arrest?**

25-50mg/kg IV/IO.

○   **How soon after the administration of a medication should you shock?**

Between 30-60 seconds. Elevate the limb (if used) in which you injected the medication and perform CPR to distribute the drug prior to shocking.

○   **If VF is terminated but then recurs, at what energy level should you defibrillate?**

At the energy level that previously resulted in successful defibrillation.

○   **While pumping, puffing, zapping, and drugging, you should be thinking about the possible causes of VF/VT. What eight causes are listed in the AHA 2000 guidelines? Hint: four Hs and four Ts.**

Hypoxemia
Hypovolemia
Hypothermia
Hyper/hypokalemia and metabolic disorders
Tamponade
Tension pneumothorax
Toxins/poisons/drugs

Thromboembolism

○   **What is the relationship between paddle size and impedance?**

The larger the size, the lower the impedance.

○   **What is the optimal paddle size?**

The largest size that allows good chest contact over the entire paddle surface area and good separation between the two paddles.

○   **Up to what age should infant paddles (4.5cm) be used?**

Up to approximately one year of age or 10kg. Above this age and weight, adult paddles should be used.

○   **Why should bare paddles not be used?**

They result in very high impedance.

○   **What should be used to help reduce impedance?**

Electrode cream or paste, saline-soaked gauze pads or self-adhesive defibrillation pads.

○   **Why should alcohol pads be avoided?**

They are a fire hazard and can produce serious chest burns.

○   **T/F: Sonographic gel is an acceptable alternative to defibrillation pads.**

False, it is not acceptable.

○   **Why must the interface medium under one electrode paddle not come into contact with the interface medium under the other electrode paddle?**

Bridging will occur, creating a short circuit and an inadequate amount of current will traverse the heart.

○   **How must electrode paddles be positioned?**

So that the heart is between them.

○   **What is theoretically the ideal paddle position?**

Anterior-posterior.

○   **Why is the anterior-posterior position impractical?**

It would interfere with CPR.

○   **What is the standard paddle position?**

One paddle is placed on the upper right chest below the clavicle and the other to the left of the left nipple in the anterior axillary line.

○   **What position should be used if dextrocardia is present?**

The mirror position of the standard.

○   **When might the anterior-posterior position be necessary?**

In an infant when only adult paddles are available.

○   **What is the proper procedure for clearing the area prior to defibrillation?**

Before each defibrillation attempt, the person who controls the defibrillator discharge buttons should state clearly, "I am going to shock on three. One—I am clear." The operator checks to make sure that there is no contact with the patient, stretcher or equipment other than the paddle handles. The operator then states, "Two—you are clear," and checks to make sure that no other personnel are in contact with the patient, including healthcare providers performing ventilations and compressions. Finally, the operator states, "Three—everybody is clear," and discharges the defibrillator.

○   **May the airway person continue to hold the BVM during defibrillation?**

No, all hands must be removed from all equipment in contact with the patient, including the endotracheal tube, ventilation bag and intravenous solutions.

○   **T/F: At the very low defibrillation dose settings required for infants, stored and delivered energies are usually identical.**

False. At these settings they may vary significantly.

○   **What special measures should be taken to ensure accurate defibrillation dosing in infants and children?**

Defibrillators should be checked at very low energy doses so that any variations between set and delivered energies could be prominently posted on the machine.

○   **A code is called in the trauma room of your ED. A ten-year-old child has become unresponsive and VF is observed on the ECG monitor. The patient is being effectively ventilated with 100% oxygen and chest compressions are being performed. You are in charge of defibrillating. What do you do first?**

Turn on the defibrillator. The synchronous mode should not be activated.

○   **What should be done next?**

Apply conductive medium to the paddles.

○   **Then what?**

Select the proper energy and charge the capacitor.

○   **What next?**

Have compressions stopped, place paddles, and recheck rhythm and patient.

○   **And now?**

Clear the area properly, apply firm pressure and defibrillate.

○   **What now?**

Reevaluate ECG and patient.

○   **What is electromechanical dissociation (EMD)?**

Electromechanical dissociation is a form of pulseless electrical activity (PEA) characterized by organized electrical activity on ECG but with inadequate cardiac output and absent pulses.

○   **What are the possible causes of EMD?**

Hypoxemia, severe acidosis, hypovolemia, tension pneumothorax, pericardial tamponade, hyperkalemia, profound hypothermia and drug overdoses.

○   **What are the most common drugs that can cause EMD?**

Tricyclic antidepressants, beta-blockers, and calcium channel blockers.

○   **What is the priority in treating EMD?**

Identification and treatment of the cause.

○   **In pediatric pulseless arrest that is not VF/VT, what is the treatment?**

CPR, epinephrine, correct the cause.

○   **T/F: The possible causes of non-VF/VT pulseless arrest are the same as those for VF/VT.**

True. Remember the four Hs and four Ts. If you can't remember them by now, hit your head against the wall three times and try again.

❍   **What should you do while trying to figure out the cause?**

Chest compressions, ventilation using 100% oxygen, intubation and administration of epinephrine.

❍   **What is an Automated External Defibrillator (AED)?**

Automated external defibrillators are external defibrillators that incorporate a rhythm analysis system and are commonly used in adults.

❍   **Do AEDs have paddles like manual defibrillators?**

No, they use two adhesive pads that are placed on the patient's chest wall and attached to the AED unit by a cable.

❍   **What two functions are served by the adhesive pads?**

They capture the surface electrocardiogram, transmitting it through the cables to the AED unit, where it is analyzed. If a defibrillation shock is indicated, the pads provide the contact to deliver the shock to the patient.

❍   **What is a fully automated AED?**

A fully automated unit requires only that the operator apply the electrodes and turn the unit on. If the victim's rhythm is determined to be either ventricular tachycardia above a present rate or ventricular fibrillation, the unit will charge its capacitors and deliver a shock.

❍   **How does a semi-automated unit differ from one fully automated?**

It requires additional operator steps, including pressing an "analyze" button to initiate rhythm analysis and pressing a "shock" button to deliver the shock. Semi automated devices use voice prompts to assist the operator.

❍   **What shock level is delivered by most AEDs?**

200 J, although some devices have a switch to enable delivery of an alternative smaller shock (e.g. 50 J).

❍   **Can AEDs be used in pediatric arrest?**

Because current units have been developed for adults, they may be considered when the child is 8 years old or older. At this age the child weights approximately 25-30kg, so that a shock of 200 J would likely deliver a defibrillating dose of approximately 8 J/kg.

❍   **In a child 8 years old or older in cardiac arrest, what do you do until the AED arrives?**

CPR.

○   **T/F: Always attach the patches to the patient before turning on the power to an AED.**

False, always turn on the power first.

○   **After 3 shocks or after any "no shock indicated," what should you do?**

Check for signs of circulation.

○   **If, after checking for signs of circulation, there is no pulse, what do you do?**

Resume CPR for one minute.

○   **After one minute of CPR, what do you do?**

Check for signs of circulation.

○   **If there are no signs of circulation, what do you do?**

Press analyze and attempt defibrillation up to three times.

○   **If there are signs of circulation, but absent or inadequate ventilation, what should you do?**

Ventilate at a rate of one breath every 5 seconds.

○   **When is noninvasive (transcutaneous) pacing indicated in children?**

In cases of profound symptomatic bradycardia refractory to BLS and ALS.

○   **T/F: Transcutaneous pacing has been shown to be effective in improving the survival rate of children with out-of-hospital unwitnessed cardiac arrest.**

False. It has not been shown to be effective.

○   **Under what weight should pediatric pacing electrodes be used?**

Under 15 kg.

○   **Where should pacing electrodes be placed on the patient prior to initiating external pacing?**

The negative electrode is placed over the heart on the anterior chest and the positive electrode behind the heart on the back. If the back cannot be used, the positive electrode is placed on the right side of the anterior chest beneath the clavicle and the negative electrode on the left side of the chest over the fourth intercostal space, in the midaxillary area.

○   **Is precise placement of electrodes necessary to effective pacing?**

No, provided that the negative electrode is placed near the apex of the heart.

○   **What types of pacing may be provided noninvasively?**

Either ventricular fixed-rate or ventricular-inhibited pacing.

○   **T/F: If smaller electrodes are used the pacemaker output required to produce capture generally will be lower than if larger electrodes are used.**

True.

○   **How must pacemaker sensitivity be adjusted if ventricular-inhibited pacing is performed?**

It must be adjusted so that intrinsic ventricular electrical activity is appropriately sensed by the pacemaker.

○   **Why is it difficult to determine if ventricular capture and depolarization are taking place?**

Because of the large pacing artifact that often occurs with transcutaneous pacing.

○   **In this circumstance, how can you determine ventricular capture and depolarization?**

By palpating a pulse or from the pressure wave of an indwelling arterial cannula.

○   **You are at the triage desk when mom brings in her three-month old. She states her daughter has had a fever for two days and is not feeding well. Patient is conscious and alert, skin is warm and dry. P 180, R 34, T 38, BP 88/62, SAT 98%. You place the child on a cardiac monitor and this is what you see. What is this rhythm?**

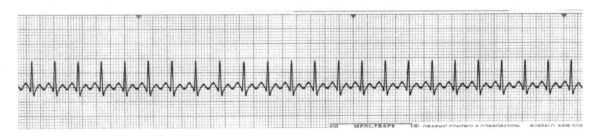

Sinus tachycardia at a rate of 180.

○   **What are the most likely causes of this rhythm?**

Fever, anxiety, dehydration.

○   **You are called to Room Eight to evaluate a three-week old infant. The child is conscious and alert, skin is cool, mottled and dry, capillary refill is delayed, R 64 and gasping, P 80, BP 60/40, SaO$_2$ 84%. The monitor shows the following rhythm. What is it?**

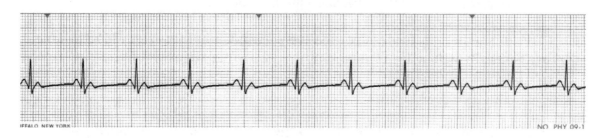

Sinus bradycardia.

○   **What is the probable etiology of this rhythm?**

Hypoxia.

○   **What is the immediate treatment priority?**

Administer 100% oxygen by non-rebreather mask. Assist ventilations with BVM as necessary.

○   **You are dispatched to the scene of a high school basketball game for a player down. When you arrive, you find a fifteen-year-old player on the court. CPR is being performed by bystanders. You place your paddles in "quick look" mode and this is what you see. What is this rhythm?**

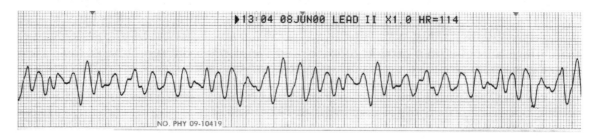

Coarse ventricular fibrillation.

○   **What immediate action must you take?**

Three rapid, stacked shocks.

⭕ **After the third shock, the patient converts to the following rhythm. What is it?**

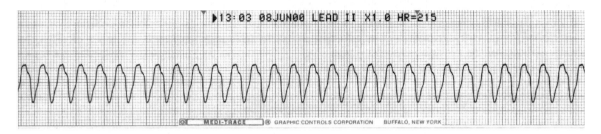

Ventricular tachycardia.

⭕ **What do you do now?**

Check for a pulse. If no pulse, defibrillate. If pulse, cardiovert.

⭕ **There is no pulse and you defibrillate at 360 joules. The patient converts to the following rhythm. What is it?**

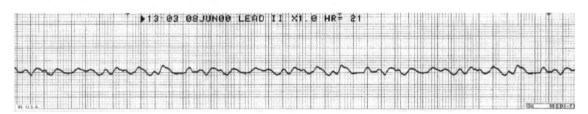

Fine ventricular fibrillation.

⭕ **What now?**

Defibrillate and 360 joules.

⭕ **You defibrillate at 360 joules and the patient converts to the following rhythm. What is it?**

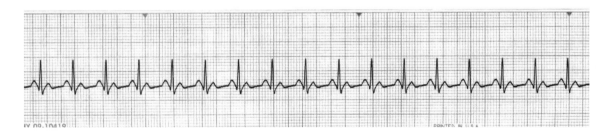

For a fifteen year-old, this would be a sinus tachycardia if accompanied by a pulse. If no pulse, pulseless electrical activity (PEA).

❍   **Dad brings in his eight year-old son, who is conscious, alert and oriented. Dad states he was playing baseball with his son in the yard, who suddenly felt weak and dizzy. He had him rest and drink some water, but the symptoms persisted, so he brought him to the emergency department. Skin is warm and dry, PERRL, P 280, R 22, BP 110/72, SaO$_2$ 99%. The monitor shows the following rhythm. What is it?**

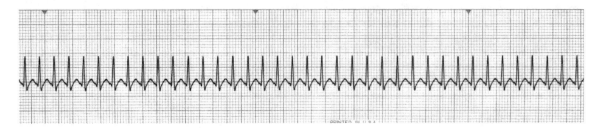

Supraventricular tachycardia.

❍   **What should you do?**

As the patient is currently stable, obtain detailed history and physical, monitor closely, establish IV access, and administer adenosine 0.1 mg/kg rapid IVP followed by a 5 ml saline flush. Call for a cardiology consult.

❍   **While waiting for the cardiologist, the patient lapses into unconsciousness. What should you do?**

Immediate cardioversion.

❍   **If you saw this rhythm on the monitor but there was no pulse, what algorithm would you follow?**

The pulseless arrest algorithm.

TRAUMA RESUSCITATION

"Anger, if not restrained, is frequently more hurtful to us than injury that provokes it."
~ Seneca ~

"Rapid cardiorespiratory assessment and prompt establishment of effective ventilation, oxygenation, and perfusion are the keys to the successful treatment of a child with a life-threatening illness or injury. The purpose of this chapter is to present those principles of care that impact the integrity of the airway, breathing and circulation or influence the priorities of advanced life support (ALS) for the pediatric trauma patient."

○ **What two courses are recommended by PALS for information about the fundamentals of pediatric trauma management?**

The Advanced Trauma Life Support Course (ATLS) of the American College of Surgeons and the Advanced Pediatric Life Support Course (APLS) of the American Academy of Pediatrics and the American College of Emergency Physicians.

○ **What is the leading cause of death and disability in the pediatric age group?**

Trauma.

○ **T/F: Injured children have a significant potential for full recovery.**

True.

○ **When should resuscitation begin after an injury?**

As soon as possible, preferably at the scene.

○ **How do the principles of resuscitation differ in the seriously injured child from any other pediatric patient?**

In general, they don't. However, some aspects of initial stabilization of the pediatric trauma patient are unique and require special emphasis.

○ **What are two fundamental aspects of the primary survey in an injured child?**

Assessment and support of cardiopulmonary function are fundamental aspects of the primary survey performed during the initial minutes of trauma care.

❍   **Why must a rapid thoracoabdominal examination be performed during the primary survey?**

To detect life-threatening chest or abdominal injuries or conditions that may interfere with successful resuscitation.

❍   **When would you perform needle decompression of tension pneumothorax, apply direct pressure control of external hemorrhage, or perform nasogastric tube decompression of gastric distention during a resuscitation?**

During the primary survey.

❍   **What is the secondary survey?**

A detailed head-to-toe examination for detection of specific injuries. The secondary survey is unique to trauma care and is not included in the PALS course.

❍   **T/F: Improper resuscitation has been identified as a major cause of preventable pediatric trauma death.**

True.

❍   **What are the three most common failures in pediatric trauma resuscitation?**

Failure to open and maintain an airway
Failure to provide appropriate fluid resuscitation
Failure to recognize and treat internal hemorrhage

❍   **At what point should a qualified surgeon be involved in pediatric trauma care?**

As early as possible in the course of resuscitation.

❍   **Which pediatric trauma patients should be transported to trauma centers with expertise in treating pediatric patients?**

Children with multisystem trauma or significant mortality risk.

❍   **How can significant mortality risk be defined?**

Pediatric Trauma Score of 8 or less or Revised Trauma Score of 11 or less.

❍   **What special consideration must be taken in opening the airway of a multisystem trauma victim?**

Control of the cervical spine.

❍   **Why is the pediatric airway difficult to control?**

It is narrow and easily obstructed by foreign matter such as blood, mucus, and dental fragments.

❍   **What are the two primary techniques for clearing the pediatric airway of foreign matter?**

Suctioning with a rigid, large-bore device, such as a Yankauer suction catheter and, occasionally, direct foreign-body retrieval with Roverstein (pediatric Magill) forceps.

❍   **T/F: Cervical spine injury is less common in pediatric than adult trauma.**

True, because the child's spine is more elastic and mobile than that of the adult, and the softer pediatric vertebrae are less likely to fracture with minor stress.

❍   **T/F: The risk of cervical spine injury is increased whenever a child is subjected to the inertial forces applied to the neck during acceleration-deceleration.**

True, because the child's head is proportionally larger than the head of an adult and is more likely to "lead" if the child falls or is propelled through or out of an automobile.

❍   **Spinal cord damage secondary to acceleration-deceleration injury is usually secondary to what spinal injury?**

Subluxation, most often at the atlantooccipital base (base of skull-C1) or atlantoaxial (C1-C2) joints in infants and toddlers or the lower (C5-C7) cervical spine in school-age children.

❍   **What are the two main categorizations of spinal cord injury?**

Anatomical and functional.

❍   **What is anatomical spinal cord injury?**

That associated with bony vertebral abnormality.

❍   **What is functional spinal cord injury?**

Spinal cord injury without radiographic abnormality (SCIWORA).

❍   **What is it about the pediatric spine that permits SCIWORA?**

Its increased elasticity and mobility caused by relative laxity of the cervical spine ligaments, incomplete development of the cervical musculature, and the shallow orientation of facet joints in young children.

❍   **T/F: SCIWORA accounts for a number of pre-hospital deaths that previously were attributed to head trauma.**

True.

❍   **Because of the recognition of SCIWORA as an important cause of pediatric spinal cord injury, what test used in adults to rule out injury in the cervical spine in adult blunt trauma victims cannot rule out such injury in children?**

The lateral cervical spine x-ray.

❍   **As a result of the recognition of SCIWORA, what special precautions must be taken in all children with multiple injuries, especially those who are apneic?**

Precautions to avoid potential exacerbation of cervical spine injury in each phase of airway management and control.

❍   **What three mechanisms can cause respiratory arrest from local obstruction or problems with CNS control in the child with severe closed head injury?**

Upper airway closure due to soft tissue obstruction
Cervical spine transection with subsequent respiratory arrest
Midbrain or medullary contusion

❍   **What is the primary method of maintaining an open airway during pediatric trauma resuscitation?**

Combined jaw-thrust/spinal-stabilization maneuver.

❍   **T/F: Traction must be maintained on the neck at all times.**

False. Neutral stabilization, never traction.

❍   **Why is the head tilt-chin lift maneuver contraindicated in the trauma patient?**

Manipulation of the head may result in conversion of an incomplete to a complete spinal cord transection.

❍   **At what point may an oral airway be used?**

After the airway has been effectively opened and the cervical spine has been simultaneously stabilized, an oral airway may be placed in an unconscious patient.

❍   **Why is correct semirigid extrication collar sizing important?**

Because excessively large collars may allow neck flexion or hyperextension.

○ **Why should soft collars be avoided?**

They do not immobilize the cervical spine effectively and have no role in initial stabilization of the child with potential cervical spine injuries.

○ **What equipment is needed for optimal immobilization of the cervical spine?**

Long spine board
Commercial head immobilizers, foam blocks or linen rolls
Tape
Cervical collar

○ **Other than size, why are adult spine boards inappropriate for use in children?**

Because the prominent occiput of the child causes the neck to flex when the child is placed on a completely flat spine board.

○ **Other than size, what is the difference between a pediatric and an adult spine board?**

The pediatric spinal board has shallow head wells to facilitate the maintenance of neutral position.

○ **If a pediatric spine board is not available, how can you alter an adult board for a child?**

Place a thin layer of firm padding under the child's torso (shoulders) to elevate it approximately 2 cm, allowing the head to assume a neutral position.

○ **What are the five indications for endotracheal intubation of the child trauma victim?**

Respiratory failure/arrest
Airway protection
Airway obstruction
Coma
Need for prolonged ventilatory support or neurological resuscitation

○ **How is respiratory failure defined?**

Hypoventilation, arterial hypoxemia despite supplemental oxygen therapy, and/or respiratory acidosis.

○ **How is coma defined in children?**

Glasgow Coma or modified Pediatric Coma Score of 8 or less.

❍   **Why is endotracheal intubation of the pediatric trauma victim more difficult than in the medical patient?**

The neck must remain in a neutral position and cannot be hyperextended during the procedure.

❍   **Why is the nasotracheal route contraindicated in children less than 8 years of age?**

Because it is extremely difficult to direct the tube anteriorly through the vocal cords in young children without direct visualization. In addition, adenoid tissue is much more prominent and susceptible to injury during emergency intubation.

❍   **Under what circumstance can endotracheal intubation by one person be accomplished in the trauma victim?**

If the child is properly immobilized on a spine board and a semirigid cervical collar is in place.

❍   **What is the role of the second rescuer in endotracheal intubation in trauma?**

One rescuer must stabilize the neck.

❍   **What procedure may precede intubation?**

Bag-valve-mask ventilation and oxygenation.

❍   **If the child is conscious, what should be done prior to intubation to avoid increasing intracranial pressure?**

Administration of a short-acting neuromuscular blocking agent followed immediately by a sedative or anesthetic and lidocaine.

❍   **What is important to determine prior to administration of blocking agents and sedatives?**

The child's neurological and cardiovascular status.

❍   **What is the main contraindication to the use of some sedatives?**

Hypotension.

❍   **Use of blocking agents and sedatives should be limited to which personnel?**

Only those who are familiar with their use and complications and are properly trained in the technique of rapid sequence induction.

❍   **What are the 11 steps for rapid sequence intubation?**

Brief medical history and physical assessment
Preparation of equipment, personnel, medications
Monitoring
Preoxygenation
Premedication
Cricoid Pressure
Sedation
Paralysis
Intubation
Postintubation observation and monitoring
Continued sedation and paralysis

○   **What two drugs can be used to inhibit the bradycardic response to hypoxemia during RSI?**

Atropine and glycopyrrolate.

○   **T/F: Cricothyrotomy is commonly used to control the pediatric airway.**

False. It is rarely necessary.

○   **When may cricothyrotomy be required?**

In the presence of orofacial trauma.

○   **What recent development has reduced the need for cricothyrotomy?**

The increasing availability of fiberoptic laryngoscopy.

○   **What are the physical indicators of effective respiratory effort?**

Adequate bilateral, symmetrical chest rise and air entry with no central cyanosis.

○   **How should an injured child with adequate ventilation receive supplemental oxygen?**

In the highest available concentration through a nonrebreathing mask.

○   **What should you do if respiratory effort is ineffective?**

Assist ventilations with a bag-valve-mask device and reservoir delivering 100% oxygen.

○   **What is associated with respiratory acidosis secondary to injury?**

Alveolar hypoventilation.

○   **What type of acidosis is caused by hypovolemia and shock?**

Metabolic.

O   **How can hyperventilation affect metabolic acidosis?**

By temporarily buffering it.

O   **What cerebral advantage may hyperventilation have?**

It may reduce the increased intracranial pressure if cerebral carbon dioxide vascular reactivity is preserved.

O   **Why should extreme hyperventilation be avoided?**

It may reduce cerebral blood flow to levels associated with ischemia.

O   **What factors can compromise ventilation of the injured child?**

Gastric distention and leak around an uncuffed endotracheal tube.

O   **When should you insert a nasogastric tube?**

After the airway has been secured.

O   **When should a nasogastric tube be avoided?**

In children with severe craniofacial trauma with maxillofacial or basilar skull fracture to avoid potential intracranial placement of nasogastric tubes.

O   **What are the four elements of circulatory support in pediatric trauma?**

Control of external hemorrhage
Assessment and support of cardiovascular function and systemic perfusion
Restoration and maintenance of adequate blood volume
Surgical intervention to control internal bleeding

O   **What is thought to be the leading cause of preventable death in children with multiple injuries?**

Failure to recognize and control internal bleeding.

O   **Why is blood transfusion of paramount importance in the initial stabilization of the pediatric trauma patient who has sustained significant blood loss?**

To restore oxygen delivery as well as intravascular volume.

O   **How do you accomplish the immediate control of external hemorrhage?**

Direct pressure with a gloved hand over the wound using sterile gauze dressings.

❍ **Why are these dressings applied with pressure more effective than bulky dressings?**

Bulky dressings may absorb large quantities of blood and may dissipate the amount of pressure actually applied to the wound.

❍ **When should the blind application of hemostats be used?**

They shouldn't.

❍ **When should tourniquets be used?**

Only in cases of traumatic amputation associated with uncontrolled bleeding from a major vessel.

❍ **Above what percentage of blood volume loss will signs of shock be observed?**

15%.

❍ **After what percentage of blood loss will hypotension be present?**

After 25%-30% or more of the child's blood volume has been lost acutely.

❍ **T/F: Signs of shock may initially be subtle in the child and may be difficult to differentiate from signs of pain or fear.**

True.

❍ **What are the early signs of circulatory failure?**

Tachycardia
Decrease in intensity of peripheral pulses
Delayed capillary refill

❍ **What number and kind of IV catheter should be used in pediatric trauma?**

Two short, large-bore catheters.

❍ **Are the upper or lower extremities preferred, and why?**

The upper extremities, because injuries to the lower extremities are more common in young children.

❍ **Is the efficacy of fluid resuscitation in young subjects related more to site of venous access, or fluid volume, type, and speed of delivery?**

Volume, type and speed.

❍   **What route should be used if intravenous access cannot be established?**

Intraosseous.

❍   **If you are unable to establish intravenous or intraosseous access, what should you do?**

Attempt percutaneous cannulation of the femoral vein at the groin or saphenous vein cutdown at the ankle if skilled personnel are available.

❍   **Fill in the blanks: healthcare providers should attempt to secure the _____ catheter in the _____ vein possible at the sites with which they are most _____.**

Healthcare providers should attempt to secure the <u>largest</u> catheter in the <u>largest</u> vein possible at the sites with which they are most <u>experienced</u>.

❍   **Define compensated shock.**

Systemic perfusion is inadequate but blood pressure is normal.

❍   **What class of hemorrhage is present in compensated shock?**

Class I-II, mild to moderate hypovolemia.

❍   **How should compensated shock be treated?**

With rapid volume replacement with a bolus of 20 ml/kg of isotonic crystalloid solution.

❍   **What two isotonic crystalloids are used in resuscitation?**

Normal saline and lactated ringers.

❍   **When should you consider administration of blood?**

If signs and symptoms of shock persist after two or three boluses of crystalloid solution.

❍   **What class of hemorrhage is uncompensated shock?**

Class III-IV.

❍   **What percentage of blood loss results in uncompensated shock?**

25%-30%.

❍   **What is the immediate treatment for uncompensated shock?**

Immediate volume replacement and blood transfusion.

○   **How should these fluids be administered?**

Using a pressure infusion system or "wide open" intravenous system may be necessary.

○   **When should urgent transfusion and possibly surgery be considered?**

If the child fails to respond to the administration of two or three boluses of crystalloid solution (approximately 40-60 ml/kg).

○   **What type of blood transfusion should be given in shock?**

Packed red blood cells mixed with normal saline warmed to body temperature.

○   **What is the initial dose?**

10 ml/kg.

○   **What should you use if packed red cells are not available?**

Whole blood.

○   **What is the initial dose?**

20 ml/kg.

○   **How many times should you repeat these doses?**

Until systemic perfusion is adequate.

○   **T/F: Administered blood should always be type specific and crossmatched.**

False. Transfusions must not be delayed to await compatibility studies if shock continues despite crystalloid therapy. Instead, O-negative blood should be administered immediately.

○   **What is indicated if shock persists despite control of external hemorrhage and volume resuscitation?**

Internal bleeding.

○   **What is the treatment if internal hemorrhage is suspected?**

Continued transfusion therapy, surgical assessment, and probable urgent surgical exploration.

○   **What can the trauma team do to ensure early surgical intervention?**

Notify a qualified surgeon before the arrival of any child with multiple injuries in the emergency department so that the surgeon may be involved in initial evaluation and stabilization. Blood samples for type and crossmatch should also be obtained immediately upon the arrival of a child in the emergency department.

○ **T/F: Volume resuscitation should be limited in a child with head injury.**

False. Volume resuscitation and blood transfusion should continue as long as signs of shock are present in a child with head injury.

○ **Won't volume resuscitation increase the likelihood of cerebral injury in head trauma?**

No, ischemia may complicate traumatic brain injury unless intravascular volume is effectively restored.

○ **What are the dangers of excessive fluid resuscitation?**

Complications of hypervolemia or extravascular fluid shifts.

○ **T/F: Isolated head injury can cause sufficient blood loss to produce shock in a child.**

True, isolated head injury rarely causes shock but may if bleeding scalp lacerations are not appropriately managed.

○ **What should be suspected if shock is present in a child with head injury and no external bleeding?**

An internal bleeding source: intra-abdominal hemorrhage must be ruled out.

○ **What are three signs of intra-abdominal bleeding caused by organ rupture?**

Abdominal tenderness
Distention that does not improve following nasogastric decompression
Signs of shock

○ **What nasogastric findings support the diagnosis of organ rupture?**

Aspirate that is blood stained.

○ **What is the role of military antishock trousers (MAST) in the treatment of hemorrhagic shock in children?**

Unclear – there is no population of pediatric patient in which use of the MAST has been shown to improve survival. They may have some role in stabilization of long bone or pelvic fractures.

○   **What serious complications can result from the use of MAST?**

Compartment syndrome or ischemia to the limbs or respiratory failure cause by inflation of the abdominal compartment impeding diaphragmatic excursion.

○   **What is thought to cause the rise in blood pressure following MAST inflation?**

Increased vascular resistance produced by obstruction of lower extremity blood flow, rather than augmented venous return.

○   **Why is this not a good thing?**

There is concern that this may increase the rate of bleeding in areas above the garment and worsen survival, particularly in penetrating trauma.

○   **What is the current thinking on MAST in pediatric patients?**

While anecdotal reports suggest that MAST my occasionally be useful in the management of shock associated with pediatric blunt trauma if vascular access is delayed, recent evidence indicates that the trousers offer no demonstrable survival benefit for most children with profound hypotension and may actually worsen outcome in children with mild to moderate hypotension. Thus, MAST cannot be recommended for use in the treatment of hemorrhagic shock associated with major pediatric trauma, except in cases involving unstable pelvic fractures.

○   **If used in children with unstable pelvic fractures, what is the minimum pressure to which MAST should be inflated?**

40-50 mmHg.

○   **What should be done if the patient's condition deteriorates suddenly after MAST inflation?**

The device should be deflated immediately.

○   **When should the abdominal compartment be inflated?**

It should never be inflated, because it may compress abdominal contents against the diaphragm and compromise ventilation.

○   **Why is severe head injury no longer considered a contraindication to MAST?**

The trousers produce minimal increase in intracranial pressure.

○   **Which routes of IV access are limited by MAST?**

The femoral and intraosseous routes, although infusion of fluid and drugs from more distal sites does not appear to be hindered by MAST inflation.

❍   **T/F: Serious chest injuries are common in pediatric trauma.**

False, they are uncommon.

❍   **What types of intrathoracic injuries constitute an immediate threat to life.**

Tension pneumothorax
Open pneumothorax
Massive hemothorax
Cardiac tamponade
Flail chest

❍   **Why is it more likely to find severe intrathoracic injury without chest wall or rib injury in children than in adults?**

Because the pediatric chest wall is extremely compliant. For this reason intrathoracic injuries must be suspected and ruled out whenever there is a significant history of blunt trauma.

❍   **What is indicated by the presence of rib fractures?**

That severe chest trauma has occurred, and injury to underlying organs, such as the liver, spleen, and lungs is likely to be present.

❍   **Which two injuries are most likely to impede initial stabilization of the pediatric trauma victim?**

Tension pneumothorax and open pneumothorax.

❍   **How are flail chest and massive hemothorax best managed?**

Initially by aggressive treatment of the respiratory failure and shock they produce.

❍   **How is flail chest best managed?**

With supportive care often positive-pressure ventilation.

❍   **How is hemothorax managed?**

With urgent placement of a chest tube.

❍   **T/F: Cardiac tamponade is common in childhood blunt trauma.**

False, it is extremely rare, but requires emergent surgical drainage and repair.

❍ **What causes tension pneumothorax?**

The trapping of air behind a one-way "flap-valve" defect in the lung that results from penetrating chest trauma or acute barotrauma sustained at the moment of blunt injury.

❍ **What are the signs of a child with tension pneumothorax?**

Severe respiratory distress
Distended neck veins
Contralateral tracheal deviation
Hyperresonance, decreased chest expansion and diminished breath sounds on the side of
  injury
All of these may be difficult to assess in children

❍ **Is tension pneumothorax better detected during positive pressure ventilation or respiration?**

Positive pressure ventilation.

❍ **As tension pneumothorax progresses, what are the effects on systemic circulation?**

Systemic perfusion will be severely compromised as the mediastinum shifts to the contralateral side, twisting the superior and inferior vena cavae and obstructing venous return.

❍ **What is the treatment for tension pneumothorax?**

Needle decompression followed by placement of a chest tube.

❍ **T/F: Tension pneumothorax should be confirmed by chest x-ray prior to decompression.**

False. Decompression must precede confirmatory chest x-ray if signs of respiratory distress or shock are present.

❍ **What type of needle is used for chest decompression?**

An over-the-needle catheter.

❍ **Where is the needle inserted?**

Through the second intercostal space on the midclavicular line just above the third rib.

❍ **T/F: The needle must be attached to a one-way valve.**
False. The pneumothorax may be vented to the atmosphere until a chest tube is inserted.

○ **What is another name for open pneumothorax?**

Sucking chest wound.

○ **What causes open pneumothorax?**

A penetrating chest wound that allows free, bi-directional flow of air between the affected hemithorax and the surrounding atmosphere.

○ **How does an open pneumothorax prevent effective ventilation?**

By causing equilibration of intrathoracic and extrathoracic pressure. This results in a paradoxical shifting of the mediastinum to the contralateral side with each spontaneous breath.

○ **Why are sucking chest wounds more lethal in children than adults?**

Because the mediastinum is particularly mobile during childhood.

○ **What is the primary treatment for respiratory decompensation associated with an open pneumothorax?**

Positive pressure ventilation.

○ **What else should be done?**

The wound should be covered using an occlusive dressing such as Vaseline® gauze. This dressing should be taped on three sides to allow egress of entrapped air during exhalation. Dressing application should be followed by insertion of a chest tube, unless the defect is so large that it requires immediate surgical repair.

○ **T/F: Most pediatric trauma-related mortality occurs after admission to the hospital.**

False, it occurs prior to admission, either in the field or in the emergency department.

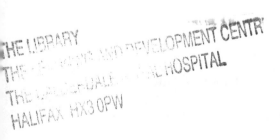

NEWBORN RESUSCITATION

"Baby: an alimentary canal with a loud voice at one end and no responsibility at the other."
~ Elizabeth Adamson ~

"Ideally, newborn resuscitation should take place in the delivery room or the neonatal ICU, because trained personnel and appropriate equipment should always be readily available in these settings . . . Unfortunately, many deliveries occur outside the delivery room—in the home, en route to the hospital, or in the emergency department—where conditions for resuscitation may be sub optimal. This chapter offers a practical approach to resuscitation of the neonate in settings other than the delivery room, so recommendations very slightly from those contained in the NRP [Neonatal Resuscitation Program]."

○ **What training program should be completed by all personnel in the delivery room, newborn nursery, and neonatal intensive care personnel who may deal with a neonate in distress?**

The Neonatal Resuscitation Program (NRP).

○ **What is the most significant physiological change undergone by the neonate?**

The transition from fetal to neonatal circulation.

○ **What system must become instantly functional in this transition?**

The respiratory system, essentially nonfunctional in utero, must suddenly initiate and maintain oxygenation and ventilation.

○ **What is required to assist the majority of term newborns in making this transition?**

Maintenance of temperature, suctioning of the airway, and mild stimulation.

○ **Of the small number of newborns that require further intervention, most respond to what?**

Administration of a high concentration of inspired oxygen and ventilation with a bag and mask.

❍　**What measure may be necessary if oxygen and bagging don't work?**

Chest compressions.

❍　**What is the least commonly required intervention in newborn resuscitation?**

Resuscitative medications.

❍　**What does the "inverted pyramid" illustrate?**

The relative frequencies and priorities of neonatal resuscitation.

❍　**What must follow each step in the pyramid to prevent unnecessary intervention and potential complications?**

Reassessment.

❍　**Why must pre-hospital delays and stops in the emergency department or admitting office be avoided?**

Because the best resuscitation results are obtained in a well-equipped and well-staffed delivery room.

❍　**In addition to a standard obstetrical tray, what other tray should every emergency department have for emergent deliveries?**

A neonatal resuscitation tray that is readily accessible and regularly checked and replenished.

❍　**In addition to appropriate equipment, what else should this tray contain?**

Charts listing correct medication doses for neonates of various weights.

❍　**What is the ideal equipment to have on hand in the emergency department to warm the neonate?**

A radiant warmer.

❍　**What should be done as soon as the need for neonatal resuscitation becomes evident?**

A prearranged plan should be activated to organize personnel according to levels of competence.

❍　**There is usually little time to obtain an in-depth obstetrical history. What minimum key history is needed?**

Particulate meconium in the amniotic fluid

Prematurity
Twins
Narcotics

○   **If there is a history of particulate meconium in the amniotic fluid, what should the resuscitation team be prepared to do?**

Suction the mouth and nose and consider suctioning of the trachea under direct visualization or newborns with no spontaneous respirations, poor tone and HR < 100 bpm

○   **If twins are anticipated, what should the resuscitation team be prepared to do?**

Resuscitate two infants.

○   **If labor is premature, what should the resuscitation team be prepared to do?**

Assist ventilations.

○   **If narcotics have been administered to the mother, or if the mother is a known drug addict, what should the resuscitation team be prepared to do?**

Assist ventilations.

○   **What three essential things may be difficult to maintain during pre-hospital neonatal transport?**

Body temperature
Airway
Vascular access

○   **What must be verified on arrival in the emergency department following a field delivery?**

Airway placement and placement of vascular catheters.

○   **Which personnel involved in a delivery and newborn resuscitation should use universal precautions?**

All personnel.

○   **When is it permissible to perform direct mouth suctioning of the neonatal trachea.**

Never.

○   **Which critical metabolic derangement can be exacerbated by hypothermia in the newborn?**

Acidosis.

❍ **What three things can you do to minimize heat loss in a neonate?**

Quickly dry the amniotic fluid covering the infant
Remove wet linens from contact with the baby
Place the infant under a preheated warmer or heat lamps

❍ **What precaution should be taken to prevent hazards to the infant when using a heating lamp?**

Be sure to maintain the recommended distance from the baby.

❍ **What alternative methods are available for warming the neonate when radiant warmers and heating lamps are not available?**

Warm blankets
Warm towels
Warming mattresses
Placement of towel-wrapped latex gloves filled with warm water around infant
Mom- if initial evaluation indicates the infant is stable it may be placed naked against the
    mother's body with covers placed over both mother and child

❍ **How should the newborn be positioned?**

On his or her back or side with the neck in a neutral position.

❍ **Why should hyperextension of the neck be avoided?**

It may produce airway obstruction.

❍ **When placing the infant on his or her back, what can you do to insure neutral position?**

A rolled blanket or towel may be placed under the back and shoulders, thus elevating the
torso 3/4 or 1 inch off the mattress to extend the neck slightly.

❍ **How should the infant be positioned if copious secretions are present?**

On his or her side with the neck slightly extended to allow secretions to collect in the
mouth rather than in the posterior pharynx.

❍ **When should the trachea be suctioned if meconium staining is observed?**

Before other resuscitative steps are taken.

❍ **If meconium is absent but suctioning is required to ensure a patent airway, should the mouth or the nose be suctioned first?**

The mouth.

❍   **What suctioning equipment should be used?**

A bulb syringe may be adequate, and mechanical suction may also be used.

❍   **What sized suction catheter should be used?**

8 or 10F.

❍   **If mechanical suction is used, what negative pressure should not be exceeded?**

-100mm Hg (-136 cm H_2O).

❍   **What negative response can be produced by deep suctioning of the oropharynx?**

A vagal response that can cause bradycardia and/or apnea.

❍   **How long should you perform suctioning?**

No longer than 3-5 seconds per attempt.

❍   **What should you monitor during suctioning?**

The infant's heart rate.

❍   **What should you do between suctioning attempts?**

Time should be allowed between suction attempts for spontaneous ventilation or assisted ventilation with 100% oxygen.

❍   **What three forms of mild stimulation will be effective in stimulating breathing in most newborns?**

Drying, warming and suctioning.

❍   **What are two additional safe methods of stimulation?**

Slapping or flicking the soles of the feet and rubbing the infant's back.

❍   **What should you do if spontaneous and effective respirations are not established after a brief period (5 to 10 seconds) of stimulation?**

Positive-pressure ventilation.

❍ **When should you begin your assessment of the newborn?**

After the infant is dried and placed in a warm environment, the airway is cleared, and stimulation is provided. These interventions should be accomplished virtually simultaneously. If delivery occurs before arrival in the emergency department, assessment should be performed immediately after the infant is placed in a warmed environment.

❍ **If respirations are deemed adequate on assessment, what should you check next?**

Heart rate.

❍ **If respirations are inadequate or gasping is present, what should you do?**

Begin positive-pressure ventilation immediately.

❍ **If respirations are shallow or slow, what should you do?**

A brief period of stimulation may be attempted while 100% oxygen is administered. The rate and depth of respirations should increase after a few seconds of stimulation and administration of oxygen.

❍ **If no response is noted after 5-10 seconds of stimulation and oxygen administration, what should you do?**

Positive-pressure ventilation with 100% oxygen should be initiated.

❍ **Why shouldn't you continue to stimulate the infant at this point?**

Continued stimulation of an obviously depressed, cyanotic and unresponsive infant increases hypoxemia and delays initiation of ventilation.

❍ **"The mere presence of respirations does not guarantee adequate ventilation." Explain.**

Shallow respirations may primarily ventilate airway dead space and thus provide inadequate alveolar ventilation, resulting in hypoxemia, hypercarbia, and slowing of the heart rate.

❍ **What vital sign is considered a reliable indicator of the newborn's degree of distress?**

Heart rate.

❍ **What three methods are used in evaluating heart rate?**

Palpation of the pulse at the base of the umbilical cord

Palpation of the brachial or femoral pulse
Auscultation of the apical heart sound with a stethoscope

○   **What are the problems associated with using a cardiotachometer monitoring system at this point?**

Time is required to set up the system and electrodes may not stick well while vernix still covers the newborn's body.

○   **What should you do if the heart rate is greater than 100 beats per minute and spontaneous respirations are present?**

Continue with the assessment.

○   **What should you do if the heart rate is less than 100 beats per minute?**

Positive-pressure ventilation with 100% oxygen should be initiated immediately.

○   **What should you do if the heart rate is less than 60 bpm and not increasing rapidly despite effective ventilation with 100% oxygen?**

Chest compressions should be initiated.

○   **T/F: An infant may be cyanotic despite adequate ventilation and a heart rate greater than 100 bpm.**

True.

○   **What should you do if central cyanosis is present in a newborn with spontaneous respirations and an adequate heart rate?**

100% oxygen should be administered until the cause of the cyanosis can be determined.

○   **What is acrocyanosis?**

Peripheral cyanosis.

○   **Should you administer oxygen to an infant with peripheral cyanosis?**

No, it is a common condition in the first few minutes of life and is not indicative of hypoxemia.

○   **What is the purpose of the Apgar scoring system?**

It enables rapid evaluation of a newborn's condition at specific intervals after birth.

○   **What are the five objective signs measured by the Apgar?**

Appearance (color)
Pulse (heart rate)
Grimace (reflex irritability)
Activity (muscle tone)
Respirations

○   **At what intervals should the Apgar be measured?**

One and five minutes of age.

○   **When should you take additional scores?**

If the five-minute Apgar score is less than 7, additional scores are obtained every five minutes for a total of twenty minutes.

○   **Can the Apgar score be used to determine the need for resuscitation?**

No. If resuscitative efforts are required, they should be initiated promptly and should not be delayed while the Apgar score is obtained.

○   **How does prematurity affect the Apgar score?**

In preterm infants the Apgar score is more likely to be affected by gestational age than asphyxia.

○   **When should you be concerned about administering 100% oxygen in newborn resuscitation?**

Never. If oxygen is needed during the resuscitation of a newborn, 100% should be used without concern for its potential hazards.

○   **T/F: Only warmed and humidified oxygen should be administered.**

False. Ideally, oxygen should be warmed and humidified, but this may not be possible in an emergency situation.

○   **What methods can be used to administer oxygen to a newborn?**

A head hood, facemask attached to a non-self-inflating ("anesthesia") bag, or by a simple mask held firmly to the infant's face with at least 5 lpm oxygen flow.

○   **What are three indications for positive-pressure ventilation?**

Apnea or gasping respirations
Heart rate less than 100 bpm
Persistent central cyanosis despite administration of 100% oxygen

○   **At what rate should you assist ventilations?**

40-60 bpm.

O **How can you determine the appropriate tidal volume for bagging a neonate?**

Begin bag-valve-mask ventilations carefully and determine visually the volume and force required to produce adequate chest expansion.

O **For most newborns, what is the initial pressure required for lung inflation?**

30-40 cm H_2O. Less pressure (20 cm H_2O) is usually required for subsequent breaths.

O **What is the best indicator of appropriate inflation pressure?**

Chest wall movement.

O **What should you do if adequate chest expansion is not achieved with initial assisted ventilation?**

The head and the facemask should be repositioned.

O **What should you do if repositioning the head and facemask fail to produce effective chest expansion?**

Suction further and increase inflation pressure.

O **What should you do if you still cannot achieve effective chest expansion and improvement in color and heart rate?**

Intubate immediately.

O **When should you insert an orogastric tube?**

If BVM positive-pressure ventilation is required for more than approximately two minutes of if gastric distention develops.

O **What size orogastric tube should be used?**

8F or 10F.

O **To what should you attach the OG tube?**

Leave open to air and periodically aspirate with a syringe.

O **At what point may you discontinue positive-pressure ventilation?**

After adequate ventilation has been established for 15-30 seconds, the heart rate is 100 bpm or higher, and spontaneous respirations are present.

❍　**Should ventilation be suddenly or gradually stopped?**

Gradual reduction in the rate and pressure of assisted ventilation will increase the stimulus for the newborn to resume spontaneous breathing. If spontaneous respirations are inadequate, assisted ventilation must continue.

❍　**Many self-inflating ventilation bags have a pop-off valve. At what pressure is this valve usually preset?**

30-45 cm H_2O.

❍　**What is the problem with the pop-off valve in neonatal resuscitation?**

The initial inflation of a newborn's lungs may require higher inspiratory pressures, and the valve may prevent effective inflation unless it is occluded. Such bags should therefore have a pop-off valve that is easily bypassed.

❍　**What size bag should be used in neonatal resuscitation?**

No larger than 750 ml.

❍　**Why?**

A larger bag makes it difficult to judge the small tidal volumes administered to neonates and may increase the risk of hyperinflation and potential barotrauma.

❍　**What is the ideal sized ventilation bag for neonatal resuscitation?**

450 ml.

❍　**What is the range of neonatal tidal volume?**

6-8 ml/kg.

❍　**What must be used in conjunction with a non-self inflating ("anesthesia") bag?**

A pressure gauge.

❍　**What is the advantage of an anesthesia bag in neonatal resuscitation?**

It enables provision of a wide range of peak inspiratory pressures and more reliable delivery of high-inspired oxygen concentration than a self-inflating bag.

❍　**What are the disadvantages of an anesthesia bag?**

Requires training and practice
Will not work without an oxygen source

Can deliver very high pressures
Requires a well-modulated flow of gas into the inlet port
Requires correct adjustment of pop-off or flow-control valves

❍   **What are the ideal features of a facemask for infants?**

Designed to fit the contours of the newborn's face and have a low dead space volume (less than 5 ml).

❍   **Why are facemasks with cushioned rims recommended?**

They facilitate creation of an effective seal between face and mask.

❍   **What should a correctly positioned and sized mask cover?**

Mouth and nose but not the eyes.

❍   **What are the three indications for endotracheal intubation?**

1. Bag-valve-mask ventilation is ineffective
2. Tracheal suctioning is required for aspiration of thick, particulate meconium in a depressed newborn
3. Prolonged positive-pressure ventilation is necessary

❍   **Should tapered tubes be used for neonates?**

No, only tubes with a uniform internal diameter.

❍   **What does the black line near the tip of the endotracheal tube indicate?**

This is the vocal cord line guide. When this guide is placed at the level of the vocal cords, the tip of the tube is likely to be positioned properly in the trachea, above the carina.

❍   **What three measures can be used to estimate tube size?**

Weight
Length
Postconceptual age

❍   **What four methods should be used to verify tube placement during resuscitation?**

1. Observation of symmetrical chest movement
2. Auscultation of equal breath sounds, heard best in the axillae, and absent gurgling sounds over the stomach
3. Observation of improvement in the neonate's color, heart rate and activity
4. Detection of exhaled carbon dioxide

❍ **How should you make the final confirmation of tube placement if the tube is to remain in place after resuscitation?**

Chest x-ray.

❍ **What are the cardiac and circulatory sequelae to asphyxia?**

Peripheral vasoconstriction
Tissue hypoxia
Acidosis
Poor myocardial contractility
Bradycardia
Cardiac arrest

❍ **What are the indications for initiating chest compressions in the neonate?**

Heart rate less than 60 bpm despite effective positive-pressure ventilation with 100% oxygen for approximately 30 seconds.

❍ **When is it appropriate to delay chest compressions in order to intubate?**

Only if you are unable to effectively ventilate with a BVM.

❍ **What is the correct compression to ventilation ratio?**

3:1.

❍ **T/F: If ventilation is achieved via a BVM, chest compressions must be briefly interrupted to allow interposition of effective ventilation.**

True. This is usually not the case in the intubated infant.

❍ **What is the preferred technique for performing chest compressions in the neonate and small infant?**

Two thumbs placed on the middle third of the sternum, with the fingers encircling the chest and supporting the back. The thumbs should be positioned side by side on the sternum just below the nipple line. If the infant is extremely small or the rescuer's thumbs are extremely large, the thumbs may have to be superimposed one on top of the other.

❍ **What anatomical feature is important to avoid when performing chest compressions, and why?**

The xiphoid portion of the sternum. May cause liver damage.

❍ **How should you perform compressions if your hands are too small to encircle the chest?**

Two finger compression with the ring and middle fingers of one hand on the sternum just below the nipple line, and the other hand supporting the newborn's back.

○   **What is the depth of neonatal compression?**

Approximately one third the anterior-posterior diameter of the chest or the depth that generates a palpable pulse.

○   **What is the rate of neonatal compressions?**

120 times per minute.

○   **T/F: The relaxation phase should be longer than the compression phase.**

False, they should both be smooth and equal.

○   **T/F: The compressing thumbs or fingers should not be lifted off the sternum during the relaxation phase.**

True.

○   **When should you cease compressions?**

When the heart rate reaches 60 or more bpm.

○   **A *rate* of compressions of 120 bpm with breaths interposed at a 3:1 ration will result in provision of how many compressions and how many breaths each minute.**

90 compressions and 30 breaths each minute.

○   **What is the most common cause of bradycardia and shock in the neonatal period?**

Profound hypoxemia.

○   **When should medications be administered in cases of bradycardia and shock?**

If, despite adequate ventilation with 100% oxygen and chest compressions, the heart rate remains less than 60 bpm.

○   **What is the preferred site for vascular access during neonatal resuscitation?**

The umbilical vein, because it is easily located and cannulated.

○   **What preparation is required prior to umbilical catheterization?**

Skin prep, draped appropriately and the cord trimmed with a scalpel blade 1 cm above the skin attachment and held firmly with a ligature to prevent bleeding.

❍ **How do you identify the umbilical vein?**

It is a thin walled single vessel. In contrast, the umbilical arteries are paired, have thicker walls, and are often constricted. The lumen of the vein is larger than that of the arteries; thus the vessel that continues to bleed after the cord is cut is usually the vein.

❍ **What size catheter should be used?**

A 3.5F or a 5F umbilical catheter.

❍ **How is the catheter prepared for insertion?**

It is flushed with heparinized saline (0.5 to 1 U/ml) and attached to a three-way stopcock.

❍ **How far should the catheter be inserted?**

So that the tip is just below the skin and blood can be readily aspirated and any air bubbles evacuated. The umbilical venous catheter is inserted only until a good blood return is obtained. This should correspond to a depth of insertion of 1 to 4 cm.

❍ **What complication can result from inserting the catheter too far?**

Advancement of the catheter tip into the portal vein or hepatic circulation. Neonatal liver injury (including hemorrhage) has been linked with the administration of hypertonic and alkaline solution (e.g., THAM or sodium bicarbonate into the portal vein, so this position of the catheter tip is avoided.)

❍ **What should be suspected if free blood return is absent?**

A wedged hepatic position.

❍ **What should you do if you suspect such wedging?**

You should withdraw the catheter to a position where blood can be freely aspirated.

❍ **How long can the umbilical catheter remain in place?**

It should be withdrawn as soon as possible after resuscitation to minimize the danger of infection or portal vein thrombosis.

❍ **What is the advantage of cannulating the umbilical artery?**

It enables monitoring of blood pressure and blood sampling for blood gas analysis and evaluation of acid-base balance.

○ **What is the disadvantage of cannulating the umbilical artery?**

It is time-consuming and more difficult than venous cannulation.

○ **What other sites of cannulation can be used?**

Peripheral veins in the extremities and scalp, although they are difficult to cannulate in neonates during resuscitation.

○ **If fluid and medications are required but umbilical venous or arterial access cannot be obtained, what should you do?**

Attempt intraosseous cannula placement, which can provide access to a noncollapsible venous plexus.

○ **Where is the intraosseous cannula inserted?**

In the medial aspect of the tibia, just inferior and medial to the tibial tuberosity on the flat surface of the proximal tibia.

○ **What route of medication administration should be used when vascular access cannot be achieved?**

Endotracheal.

○ **What two drugs can be administered to the neonate by this route?**

Epinephrine and naloxone.

○ **What dosing regimen should be used for the endotracheal route in neonates?**

The dose is 0.01 to 0.03 mg/kg or 0.1 to 0.3 ml/kg IV every 3 to 5 minutes. The drug should be diluted to a volume of 3-5 ml of normal saline (use smallest volume for smallest babies), followed by several positive-pressure ventilations.

○ **What are the indications for epinephrine in neonatal resuscitation?**

Asystole or spontaneous heart rate less than 60 bpm despite adequate ventilation with 100% oxygen and chest compressions.

○ **What is the dose?**

0.01 to 0.03 mg/kg (0.1 to 0.3 ml/kg of the 1:10,000 solution). May be repeated every 3 to 5 minutes if required.

○ **When is high dose epinephrine appropriate?**

Not currently indicated but may be considered for circumstances that suggest a catecholamine resistant condition (eq. anaphylaxis, known alpha or beta blocker overdose, or severe sepsis already treated with high dose pressors.)

○ **Do the current data support the use of high dose epinephrine in neonatal resuscitation?**

Data are inadequate at present to evaluate the efficacy of high doses of epinephrine in newborns, and the safety of these doses has not been established.

○ **What is the primary complication of high dose epinephrine in newborns?**

Prolonged hypertension, which may in turn lead to complications such as intracranial hemorrhage in preterm infants.

○ **What is the endotracheal dose of epinephrine in newborns?**

The same as the IV dose – 0.01 to 0.03 mg/kg.

○ **What is the indication for volume expanders?**

Hypovolemia.

○ **What are the three primary signs of hypovolemia?**

Pallor that persists despite oxygenation
Faint pulses with a good heart rate
Poor response to resuscitation, including effective ventilation

○ **What are the three primary volume expanders for neonates?**

O-negative blood crossmatched with mother's blood
5% albumin/saline solution or other plasma substitute
Normal saline or Ringers lactate

○ **What is the dosage for volume expanders in neonatal resuscitation?**

10 ml/kg. Reassess and administer additional boluses as needed.

○ **What is naloxone?**

A narcotic antagonist that does not produce respiratory depression.

○ **What are the indications for naloxone in neonatal resuscitation?**

For the reversal of neonatal respiratory depression induced by narcotics administered to the mother within 4 hours of delivery.

❍ **What must be provided before the administration of naloxone?**

Prompt and adequate ventilatory support.

❍ **Why is continued surveillance of the infant necessary after the administration of naloxone?**

Because the duration of action of narcotics may exceed that of naloxone, and repeat administration of naloxone is often needed.

❍ **What side effects are associated with naloxone?**

It can induce a withdrawal reaction in an infant of a narcotic-addicted mother, and should be used with caution if this condition is suspected. Prolonged ventilatory support may be required by these patients.

❍ **What is the dosing of naloxone?**

0.1 mg/kg. The initial does may be repeated every 2 to 3 minutes as needed.

❍ **What are the routes of administration for naloxone?**

Intravenous, intraosseous, via the endotracheal tube, subcutaneous, or intramuscular (if perfusion is adequate).

❍ **In addition to epinephrine and naloxone, what other drugs are useful in neonatal resuscitation?**

None. There is no evidence that atropine, calcium, or sodium bicarbonate is beneficial in the acute phase of neonatal resuscitation at delivery. Sodium bicarbonate should not be used during brief resuscitation episodes, but may be beneficial when other therapies are ineffective and resuscitation is prolonged.

❍ **What problems can be caused by meconium aspiration?**

Respiratory distress
Hypoxemia
Aspiration pneumonia
Pneumothorax
Persistent pulmonary hypertension

❍ **What percentage of all deliveries are complicated by the presence of meconium in the amniotic fluid?**

Approximately 12%.

❍ **What is the consistency of amniotic fluid containing meconium?**

Thin and watery or thick and particulate, resembling pea soup.

O   **How should delivery be altered if meconium staining is detected during delivery?**

Delivery should occur in stages to enable suctioning of the newborn's pharynx before the first breath.

O   **When should the baby be suctioned?**

As soon as the head is delivered.

O   **What should you suction?**

Mouth, nose and posterior pharynx.

O   **What size suction catheter should you use?**

12F or 14F.

O   **What should you do if a large bore catheter is not available?**

Use a bulb syringe.

O   **Why must you perform suctioning before delivery of the shoulders and thorax?**

In order to decrease the risk of meconium aspiration syndrome.

O   **Meconium is found in the trachea of what percent of newborns with meconium staining despite suctioning?**

20-30%.

O   **What does this data suggest?**

That there is a significant incidence of intrauterine aspiration.

O   **When thick meconium is present, what should you do after suctioning and delivery?**

If the infant is depressed (poor tone, heart rate <100 bpm) then the infant is placed in the prepared warmed environment, and before the usual initial steps, the hypopharynx is visualized with a laryngoscope and any residual meconium is removed with suctioning The trachea is then intubated and the lower airway is suctioned. These interventions should not be delayed while the infant is dried.

O   **T/F: Suction should be applied directly to the endotracheal tube.**

True.

○   **How is this accomplished?**

With a meconium aspirator.

○   **How high should you set the suction?**

No higher than 100 mmHg.

○   **What should you do if there is a significant amount of meconium?**

Repeat intubation and suction while withdrawing the ET tube, until the aspirated material is clear or until the heart rate indicates that resuscitation should proceed without delay.

○   **What should you do if the patient's condition rapidly deteriorates before all meconium is removed?**

When an infant's condition is unstable, it may not be possible to clear the trachea of all meconium before positive-pressure ventilation must be initiated.

○   **Why should an orogastric tube be placed in these infants?**

To empty the stomach, since it may contain meconium that could later be regurgitated and aspirated.

○   **What three major risk categories are associated with the resuscitation of preterm newborns?**

Respiratory depression
Hypothermia
Intracranial bleeds

○   **Why are preterm infants more likely to become hypothermic?**

Because their ratio of body surface area to volume is higher than that of full-term neonates.

○   **Why are preterm infants more subject to intracranial bleeds?**

Because the brain of the preterm infant has a fragile subependymal germinal matrix that is vulnerable to bleeding when injured by hypoxemia, rapid changes in blood pressure, or wide fluctuations in serum osmolality.

○   **Because of this increased risk of intracranial bleeding, what should be avoided in these patients?**

Administration of hyperosmolar solutions or large boluses of volume expanders.

○   **What are the three most common complications in the postresuscitation period?**

Endotracheal tube migration (including dislodgment)
Tube occlusion by mucus or meconium
Pneumothorax

○   **What is the most common cause of endotracheal tube migration?**

Neck flexion and extension.

○   **What suggests endotracheal tube malposition or obstruction?**
Decreased chest wall movement
Diminished breath sounds
Bradycardia
Decreased oxygen saturation
Hypercarbia

○   **Why is pneumothorax difficult to diagnose by auscultation?**

Because breath sounds in the newborn (also true in infants and children) are transmitted from all areas of the lung through the thin chest wall.

○   **When should you suspect pneumothorax?**

If a newborn deteriorates after an initial good response to ventilation or fails to respond to resuscitative efforts. Additional signs of pneumothorax include unilateral decrease in chest expansion, altered intensity or pitch of breath sounds, and increased resistance to hand ventilation.

○   **Once ventilation and heart rate are adequate, what are six additional postresuscitation goals of care?**

Temperature regulation
Blood glucose regulation
ABGs and control of acidosis
Vascular access
Perfusion regulation
Chest x-ray

○   **Where should neonates be treated after resuscitation?**

In a neonatal ICU.

○   **If not available in house, how should a newborn be transported to a neonatal ICU?**

By a neonatal transport team specifically trained in the care of sick newborns.

IMMEDIATE POSTARREST STABILIZATION AND SECONDARY TRANSPORT

"He that can heroically endure adversity will bear prosperity with equal greatest of the soul; for the mind that cannot be dejected by the former is not likely to be transported without the latter."
~Henry Fielding~

"Post-resuscitation care involves patient stabilization and transport to a tertiary care facility. This chapter deals with immediate post-arrest stabilization, ongoing care within the receiving facility, and care for the ill or injured child during inter-hospital transport."

O   **What are three areas of post-resuscitation care for the critically ill or injured child?**

Patient stabilization, transport to a tertiary care facility and on-going care within that facility.

O   **What are the two major goals of post-arrest stabilization and transport?**

Prevention of secondary organ injury and delivery of the patient in optimal condition to a tertiary care setting.

O   **Because infants and children often suffer recurrent hypoxemia or hypercapnia, hemodynamic instability, and altered sensorium during the immediate postresuscitation period, to where should these patients be transferred?**

A pediatric ICU for further observation, evaluation and care.

O   **Constant evaluation of a patient's respiratory status is important. List three signs that indicate a patient is breathing effectively.**

Adequate bilateral chest expansion, equal bilateral breath sounds, and an easy unlabored respiratory effort.

O   **List five signs of inadequate ventilation for a patient experiencing respiratory distress.**

Minimal or unequal chest expansion bilaterally
Inadequate or unequal breath sounds
Nasal flaring
Paradoxical movement of the chest
Use of accessory muscles of respiration

O   **What are two advantages of measuring arterial blood gases for oxygen and carbon dioxide saturation levels?**

Confirms adequate oxygenation and effective carbon dioxide elimination.

O   **List two pieces of medical equipment that can be used to monitor blood oxygenation levels.**

A pulse oximeter or a skin surface (transcutaneous) oxygen monitor.

O   **T/F: Respiratory failure can be either a cause or a result of cardiopulmonary arrest.**

True.

O   **Paramedic Robert Ruiz-Krause has just intubated an apneic child with a 4.0mm endotracheal tube. Describe the proper procedure for ensuring the endotracheal tube is properly placed in the trachea.**

The endotracheal tube must be securely taped and proper endotracheal position confirmed by clinical assessment and chest radiograph.

O   **Explain the importance of verifying proper endotracheal tube placement prior to transporting the patient.**

In addition to the patient not being properly ventilated, proper endotracheal tube position must be verified immediately before transport because recognition of tube displacement may be difficult during transport and re-intubation is often impossible.

O   **Some children may require sedation and administration of muscle relaxants to minimize the risk of endotracheal tube displacement during transport. Name three medications that are frequently used.**

Diazepam (0.1 to 0.2 mg/kg IV) and morphine sulfate (0.1mg/kg IV), Midazolam (0.1-0.2mg/kg IV/IM).

O   **What is the main advantage (or disadvantage, depending on your perspective) or Thiopental (Pentothal)?**

It is very short acting, 5-10 minutes.

❍   **What is the dosing regimen for Lidocaine in RSI?**

1-2mg/kg IV every 30 minutes.

❍   **What is the dosing regimen for ketamine is RSI?**

1-4mg/kg IV/IM every 30-60 minutes.

❍   **What is the main negative side effect of ketamine?**

Hallucinations/emergence reaction.

❍   **What is the purpose of administering Lidocaine in RSI?**

To reduce ICP.

❍   **What are the three main neuromuscular blocking agents used in RSI?**

Succinylcholine, vecuronium, rocuronium.

❍   **Of the above medications, which is depolarizing?**

Succinylcholine.

❍   **What is the dosing regimen for succinylcholine?**

1mg/kg in children, 2mg/kg in infants, IV/IM (IM dose double the IV dose).

❍   **What is the duration of succinylcholine?**

3-5 minutes.

❍   **What is the onset of action of succinylcholine?**

Very rapid.

❍   **What is the dosing regimen for vecuronium?**

0.1-0.2mg/kg IV/IM.

❍   **What is the duration of vecuronium?**

30-60 minutes.

❍   **What is the onset of action of vecuronium?**

2-3 minutes.

❍   What is the dosing regimen of rocuronium?

0.6-1.2mg/kg.

❍   **What is the duration of rocuronium?**

30-45 minutes.

❍   **What is the onset of action of rocuronium?**

Rapid.

❍   **During mechanical ventilation the effectiveness of ventilation and oxygenation must be verified using what laboratory test?**

Arterial blood gas analysis.

❍   **Your patient has been placed on a mechanical ventilator in preparation for transport. How long after the initial ventilatory settings have been made should an arterial blood gas analysis be completed?**

After ten to fifteen minutes.

❍   **When using a volume-cycled ventilator, what is the recommended tidal volume that should be delivered to the patient?**

Ten to fifteen ml/kg.

❍   **When discussing mechanical ventilators, what does the acronym PEEP stand for?**

Positive End-Expiratory Pressure.

❍   **How often should the blood pressure of a hemodynamically unstable child be assessed?**

Blood pressure should be assessed every 5 minutes until stable and every 15 minutes thereafter. Attention to the patient's heart rate must also be closely monitored.

❍   **You are the primary care nurse in charge of a two-year-old being transferred to a tertiary care facility. Records of the patient's laboratory evaluations must accompany the transport team. List the lab tests that should be completed on your patient prior to her transport.**

Lab evaluation should include serum electrolytes, calcium and glucose; hematocrit; and arterial blood gases. Additional lab tests may be necessary based on the clinical condition of the patient. All of the lab results should accompany your patient.

○   **Explain the advantage of inserting a nasogastric tube for gravity drainage.**

The tube prevents gastric distention caused by air and is particularly useful during positive-pressure ventilation.

○   **Veronica is the PICU nurse caring for an infant that weighs 8 kg. She is calculating the initial maintenance IV fluid requirements for her patient. What is the proper volume and rate of IV fluid administration for a patient smaller than 10kg?**

The proper fluid requirement in a patient smaller than 10kg is 4ml/kg per hour (e.g., the maintenance rate for an 8 kg baby is 4 ml x 8 kg = 32 ml/hour).

○   **You are the respiratory therapist who has been asked to set the initial mechanical ventilator settings for a patient who is intubated. After assessing the patient's airway you determine the tube is properly placed and the patient has normal lung compliance. What is the recommended peak inspiratory pressure and inspiratory time for this patient with normal lung compliance?**

Effective ventilation may be achieved at peak inspiratory pressures of 20 to 30 cm water and an inspiratory time of 0.5 to 1.0 second.

○   **When mechanical ventilatory support is provided for the patient with normal lungs, a respiratory rate of _____ to _____ breaths per minute is typically required for infants and a rate of _____ to _____ breaths per minute for children.**

Infants: 20 to 30 breaths per minute
Children: 16 to 20 breaths per minute

○   **During the morning pediatric rounds you and your fellow residents have been asked to explain the advantage of using neuromuscular blocking agents during mechanical ventilation of a child with air trapping. How would you answer the attending physician's question?**

The use of neuromuscular blocking agents is advisable during mechanical ventilation of the child with air trapping because the child's spontaneous respiratory effort often contributes to further airway obstruction.

○   **Cyanosis of the mucous membranes is a clear indication of what?**

Hypoxemia.

○   **List four anatomical sites where arterial blood may be obtained for gas analysis.**

Radial artery
Posterior tibial artery

Dorsalis pedis artery
Femoral artery

○   **What are your alternatives for obtaining a blood sample for gas analysis if arterial puncture is unsuccessful?**

A capillary sample may be obtained from the heel, toe, or finger after the extremity has been warmed for fifteen minutes.

○   **When a patient with lung disease is placed on a mechanical ventilator, which setting on the ventilator's control panel is often set higher than for a patient without lung disease?**

When lung disease is present, higher respiratory rates may be needed to ensure adequate ventilation.

○   **Intubation bypasses glottic function and eliminates the physiologic positive end-expiratory pressure (PEEP) created during normal coughing, talking and crying. As the respiratory therapist caring for an intubated child, what should the PEEP setting be on the ventilator to maintain adequate functional residual capacity of the lungs?**

To maintain adequate functional residual capacity, a PEEP of 2 to 4 cm water should be provided when mechanical ventilation is initiated.

○   **List two primary advantages of using noninvasive monitoring devices such as pulse oximeters, transcutaneous oxygen and carbon dioxide monitors, and exhaled carbon dioxide monitors.**

These tools are very useful because they allow continuous assessment of oxygenation, ventilation, or both.

○   **Noninvasive monitoring devices such as those referenced in the above question may provide inaccurate data as a result of what types of medical conditions or equipment problems?**

Inaccurate results may occur as a result of hypothermia, poor peripheral perfusion, or endotracheal tube obstruction or displacement.

○   **T/F: Circulatory failure may be either the cause or the result of cardiopulmonary arrest.**

True.

○   **During a lecture to a group of medical students, Dr. Elena asks you to give her one reason frequent cardiovascular assessments are important in the post-arrest patient. What might you tell her?**

Frequent cardiovascular assessments allow appropriate therapeutic interventions to be initiated before irreversible changes occur.

○   **Whenever the infant or child demonstrates circulatory or respiratory instability, what characteristics of the patient's heart must be monitored continuously until the child's condition is stable?**

The heart rate and rhythm must be monitored continuously.

○   **T/F: Hypotension is a late sign of shock and requires rapid intervention.**

True.

○   **Pediatric residents Antonio and Sam are discussing alternative methods of monitoring a patient's blood pressure than the traditional use of a B/P cuff. When intense vasoconstriction is present, Korotkoff sounds may be difficult to hear. As an experienced ER nurse under these conditions, what might you suggest to these neophytes as an alternative?**

Under these conditions systolic blood pressure may be better estimated by palpation or by the use of a Doppler device. In patients with compromised cardiovascular function, direct intra-arterial monitoring should be instituted as soon as practical.

○   **If central venous access has been established, continuous or intermittent measurement of what type of pressure may help guide fluid administration and titration of vasoactive support?**

Right heart filling.

○   **Urine output often correlates with the effectiveness of renal and systemic perfusion. What is the preferred method of monitoring urine output?**

An indwelling catheter.

○   **As an ER resident working 16 hours on the late shift you are evaluating a child with some type of circulatory instability. What blood lab tests should be included in your assessment data?**

Laboratory evaluation of the circulatory state includes arterial blood gas and pH analysis and evaluation of serum electrolytes, lactic acid, calcium, glucose, urea nitrogen, and creatinine levels.

○   **You are the flight transport RN reviewing the lab results ordered by the physician, and you notice the presence of metabolic (lactic) acidosis. What does this finding indicate to you?**

The presence of metabolic (lactic) acidosis suggests that cardiac output and oxygen deliveries are inadequate.

○   **Lt. Pete Jaegly of Engine 16 is assessing a child's level of consciousness after the child experienced a prolonged seizure. The response to stimulation is often quantified and recorded by a simple neurologic scoring system with the mnemonic AVPU. What does AVPU stand for?**

Awake
Responsive to **V**erbal stimulation
Responsive to **P**ainful stimulation
Unresponsive

○   **You are the attending physician in the ER. While evaluating a six year-old male, you observe the child has significant central nervous system depression following a fall from the front porch of his home. In addition to BLS care, what procedure should be initiated until intracranial pressure can be evaluated more thoroughly?**

If significant CNS depression is evident, the patient should be intubated and hyperventilated with the PaCO2 maintained at 30-35mm Hg until intracranial pressure can be evaluated more thoroughly.

○   **Evaluation of the renal system is extremely important in the post-arrest patient. During your patient assessment at the beginning of the 7-3 shift, you notice that your five-year-old patient's urine output for the last eight hours has been only 5ml. Is this finding significant? What does it indicate?**

Decreased urine output (less than 1 ml/kg per hour for patients up to 30 kg) may result from prerenal causes, inadequate systemic perfusion, renal ischemic damage, or a combination of these conditions.

○   **When should an orogastric or nasogastric tube be inserted into a patient, and what is its purpose?**

If bowel sounds are absent, abdominal distention is present, or the patient requires mechanical ventilation, an orogastric or nasogastric tube should be inserted to prevent or treat gastric distention.

○   **Why is blind nasogastric tube placement contraindicated in the patient with serious facial trauma?**

Intracranial tube placement may result.

○   **What four modes of transportation can be used for the inter-hospital transport of an ill or injured pediatric patient?**

Local ambulance
Mobile ICU ambulance from the receiving hospital
Helicopter

Fixed-wing aircraft

❍ **Congratulations! After months of work you have been selected to head the committee that is developing a pediatric transport system. Ideally, which institution should provide central control?**

The tertiary care facility.

❍ **What minimum qualifications should the director of the transport service have?**

Training in pediatric emergency medicine or critical care.

❍ **Should the system be local, regional or national?**

Regional.

❍ **What is the lowest level of care that should be considered acceptable in a transport team?**

The transport team should be capable of providing pediatric ALS at the referring hospital and maintaining that level of care during transport.

❍ **Which two agencies should be responsible for the establishment of well-defined protocols for specific clinical situations that arise during transport of an ill or injured child?**

The referring facility and the tertiary care unit.

❍ **What are some advantages of using a ground ambulance compared with most aircraft?**

Ground ambulances are readily available, relatively inexpensive, and spacious. They can travel in most weather conditions and can stop easily if a procedure must be performed.

❍ **While attending a public relations event, the flight team from the local pediatric hospital is asked, "What are some advantages to using a helicopter when transporting an injured or ill child?" As a senior member of the flight crew, how would you answer this question?**

Helicopter transport is fast; it allows rapid arrival at the receiving hospital, or right to the scene of an emergency. In addition, it allows the referring hospital requesting our assistance to turn care over quickly. Lastly, traffic congestion is avoided.

❍ **How often do unfavorable weather conditions prevent a helicopter transport team from responding to a request for service?**

As often as 15% of the time.

❍   T/F: Patient monitoring and therapeutic interventions are easier to perform in a fixed-wing aircraft than in a helicopter?

True.

❍   You have been given responsibility for recruitment and selection of personnel for your hospital's pediatric transport team. Where might you focus your recruiting effort?

Members of the transport team might include local EMS personnel, medical personnel from your own facility, hospital-based critical care teams that transport patients of all ages, and dedicated pediatric and neonatal transport teams from other institutions.

❍   When looking for transportation for a critically ill or injured child from one facility to another, wouldn't the logical choice be the local EMS?

No. Local EMS teams rarely have the training, experience, or equipment for long-distance transport of an ill or injured child following resuscitation.

❍   What is the advantage to the community that has a dedicated pediatric critical care transport team?

These specialized teams provide optimal transport for critically ill children and often provide continuity of care from transport to the pediatric ICU.

❍   You are a pediatrician that has just been awakened by a telephone call at 3:17am. Wave Crest Memorial Hospital is calling about your patient in their ER that is expected to require pediatric ICU admission at a neighboring facility. Would you require your patient to be transported by a pediatric transport team?

Yes. Patients requiring that level of monitoring and care on arrival likely will need such care during transport.

❍   List the responsibilities of the referring hospital before the transport team arrives.

Copy all patient records and x-rays
Obtain transport consent
Secure IV access and endotracheal tube
Stabilize cervical spine and any fractures
Prepare blood products, if indicated
Provide lab telephone number for pending lab results

❍   List all the items that should be included when doing advance preparation for inter-hospital transport.

Names and telephone numbers of pediatric tertiary care facilities

Make a list of the pediatric transport systems

List all equipment and supplies for pediatric patients that need to be added to the standard EMS equipment

Develop and distribute administrative protocols to all members involved in the transport team

○   **Why is it best to ensure that endotracheal tubes and intra-vascular lines are properly secured before transport?**

Unfortunately, vascular catheters and ET tubes frequently dislodge during transport, often because they were inadequately secured for the moving environment.

○   **What member of a patient's medical team should make the initial call to transfer the patient to another facility?**

The initial call to transfer a patient should be made by the physician to the physician that will be accepting the transferred patient.

○   **What information should be provided by the referring physician to the receiving physician?**

Vital signs, fluids and medications administered, the events surrounding the hospitalization, a brief history of the illness/accident, and current clinical status.

○   **Why should the referring physician be contacted *after* the transport is completed and who should make the call?**

The receiving physician should contact the referring physician to identify any problems and to advise the referring physician of the patient's status.

ETHICAL AND LEGAL ASPECTS OF CPR IN CHILDREN

"To revive sorrow is cruel."
~ Sophocles ~

"This chapter presents some of the general principles underlying the ethical and legal rights and duties of pediatric patients, healthcare providers, and hospitals and relates those principles specifically to CPR, highlighting aspects unique to the care of children."

❍   **How are practitioners and hospitals that provide care for children legally judged?**

By widely accepted pediatric standards of care.

❍   **What are two of the issues that complicate decision-making for the provider in cases involving minors?**

Family privacy and parental authority.

❍   **Are there any exceptions to the "informed consent" doctrine?**

Yes, consent may be implied if needed treatment is emergent or the patient's ability to make a decision is lost.

❍   **Do all states follow the same common-law definition of "informed consent"?**

No, you must strictly adhere to your state's regulations.

❍   **Does the law protect the parents in fully determining the care of their child?**

Yes, if the parents act in the best interest of the child.

❍   **T/F: "Baby Doe" cases involve ethical decisions by providers refusing to treat a child with an infectious disease.**

False. "Baby Doe" cases include decision making in cases with severely handicapped or critically ill newborns. Decisions are made by the parents and physicians involved in the child's care.

❍   **Identify one resource the provider can utilize in dealing with complex decisions surrounding the care of neonates?**

The hospital ethics committee is a valuable resource for the healthcare providers.

❍   **How can a child acquire status of an "emancipated minor"?**

Marriage, judicial decree, military service, parental consent, failure of parents to meet legal responsibilities, living apart from and being financially independent of parents, motherhood.

❍   **By what is "standard of care" measured?**

The certification level of the rescuer
The expertise level of the rescuer
The circumstances surrounding the event

❍   **An EMT responds to a call where there is a question as to the authenticity of documents stating the victim's intent to refuse CPR. The victim is in cardiac arrest. What should the EMT do?**

The practice of initiating resuscitative efforts is generally accepted. CPR may be discontinued with further authentication of the patient's wishes or with a MD order.

❍   **T/F: Under the term "vicarious liability," the team leader is responsible for the actions of others.**

False. Each team member is held responsible for his or her actions. Each team member is held to the standard of care for his or her level of training.

❍   **T/F: The Good Samaritan law protects the EMT from acts of negligence.**

False. The traditional legal concept holds the EMT to a "reasonable care" standard. The circumstances surrounding the incident are evaluated and the skill level of the rescuer is taken into consideration.

❍   **Should the first responder attempt to assess resusitability of the cardiac arrest patient and then determine whether or not to initiate CPR?**

No. First responders are encouraged to initiate CPR in the cardiac arrest victim. Currently there are no accepted criteria for immediate determination of death by first responders. There are few exceptions to this rule.

❍   **What specific criteria for brain death in children have been established and validated?**

None. There are a number of definitions used to define brain death in children. Circumstances such as hypothermia, drug use, or idiopathic causes of brain injury or insult may alter neurologic criteria determining the diagnosis of death.

○ **T/F: If the healthcare provider can safely care for the adult patient, he or she can safely care for a child.**

False. Children are different from adults. The provider must have a sound knowledge base with pediatric standards of care.

○ **Is organ donation a consideration when a child is the victim?**

Yes. If approached with respect and sensitivity, organ donation may ultimately benefit the child's family.

○ **T/F: CPR incorrectly performed in the field is the leading source of malpractice suits against pediatricians.**

False. Birth related problems are the most common malpractice suits against pediatricians.

○ **When does the legal duty to meet a "reasonable standard" of care commence for the healthcare provider?**

Once he or she performs an act that may be construed as rendering care.

○ **What form of consent traditionally applies to the emergency situation?**

Implied consent.

○ **What patient's right was defined by Cordozo?**

A patient's right to grant permission for treatment.

○ **If a healthcare provider treats a patient without first being granted permission, what may that provider be guilty of committing?**

Assault.

○ **What are the three essential operational elements of informed consent?**

A careful assessment of the patient's decision-making capacity
A judgment as to the "voluntariness" of the decisions
A determination of the nature and extent of the information to be disclosed

○ **In what three ways is patient decision-making capacity reflected?**

In his or her ability to comprehend, communicate, and appreciate the consequences of available choices.

O   **To what does "voluntariness" refer?**

The absence of internal or extrinsic pressures that may coercively restrict patient options.

O   **What does the "reasonable person" standard require physicians to disclose when obtaining informed consent from a patient?**

Those material facts concerning treatment alternatives and risks that a reasonable person would need to make an informed decision.

O   **What is "therapeutic privilege?"**

If there is strong reason to believe that the disclosure involved in obtaining informed consent may cause serious psychological harm, physicians may be excused for failing to obtain it.

O   **T/F: States vary considerably with respect to their statutory or common-law definition of informed consent.**

True.

O   **When may parents make medical decisions on behalf of their children contrary to physician advice?**

On condition they fulfill the duty to provide necessary care for minor children.

O   **When may the state assert its interests in protecting the welfare of children by invoking child protection statutes to override parental wishes?**

If parents fail to provide their children with at least a minimum standard of medical care.

O   **If a parent makes a decision on behalf of his or her child motivated by strong family convictions, can the courts interfere?**

Courts regularly uphold such interventions when parent refusals may be life threatening.

O   **What if the consequences are grave, but not life threatening?**

States have varied in their willingness to intervene in such cases, reflecting the continuing struggle to balance the rights of individual children and family privacy.

O   **Are there exemptions to child protection statutes for parents who seek non-traditional forms of treatment based on religious convictions?**

Many state child-protection statutes have included such exemptions, although the American Academy of Pediatrics has urged states to repeal such provisions.

○   **According to Congressional guidelines, under what three conditions may treatment be withheld from neonates?**

1. The infant is chronically and irreversibly comatose
2. Treatment would merely prolong dying or would not be effective in ameliorating or correcting all of the infant's life-threatening conditions
3. Treatment would be virtually futile in terms of survival and therefore inhumane

○   **T/F: The Department of Health and Human Services has construed these provisions to exclude consideration of potential "quality of life" of the affected infant.**

True.

○   **How have these guidelines affected practice?**

While many neonatologists believe that these guidelines have led to excessive treatment of hopelessly ill infants, others report that they have not affected their practice patterns.

○   **T/F: Very low birth weight infants (<750 g) who require aggressive CPR during the first days of life have a very low likelihood of survival.**

True.

○   **What is the purpose of a hospital ethics committee?**

To ensure careful consideration of the clinical and ethical issues in difficult cases.

○   **How is a "minor" defined?**

Historically, the right of self-determination is recognized at the legal age of maturity, 18 years. Below this age a patient is considered a minor.

○   **Do minors have the right to consent to medical treatment?**

Many state legislatures and courts have expanded minors' rights to consent to medical treatment, although great variability in this approach exists from state to state.

○   **What are "mature minor" rules?**

Statutory rules that uphold the validity of consent given by minors if the treatment is appropriate and the minor is considered capable of comprehending the clinical circumstances and therapeutic options.

○   **What are two conditions that some states allow minors to consent to treat?**

Venereal disease and substance abuse.

O   **What is a "variable competence approach" to minors' consent?**

One that considers developmental aspects of cognitive and psychosocial maturation.

O   **In order to prevail in a malpractice suit, what must the patient prove?**

That the healthcare provider failed in his or her *duty* to provide the patient with the degree of knowledge, skill, and care usually exercised by a reasonable and prudent provider under similar circumstances, given the prevailing state of medical knowledge and available resources, and that the *specific injury* was *caused* by that failure.

O   **Are errors in judgment evidence of malpractice?**

Not by themselves.

O   **When does a provider's legal duty toward a patient begin?**

With a mutual agreement to provide care for compensation or with any act that may represent an undertaking to provide care.

O   **Must a patient have suffered an injury in order to prevail in a malpractice suit?**

Yes. Even if evidence demonstrates that the care provided was substandard, a claim of medical malpractice will fail if the patient escaped injury.

O   **What is "standard of care"?**

The degree of care and skill expected of a reasonably competent practitioner of the same class, acting in the same or similar circumstances.

O   **What is the "strict locality rule"?**

In judging standard of care, it limits the comparison standard to the same geographic area as the defendant provider.

O   **Is the "strict locality rule" universally applied?**

No. It has been abandoned in some courts, and in some states, in favor of a more regional or national standard.

O   **T/F: Medical malpractice cases concerning CPR have been limited to in-hospital cases in which the risk of cardiac arrest could be anticipated.**

True. Successful action against laypersons that attempt out-of-hospital CPR seems unlikely.

○ **May a person trained in CPR be legally held to AHA guidelines?**

This is unclear. Some courts regard the AHA CPR guidelines as a national standard of care.

○ **T/F: Failure to obtain consent can be considered malpractice.**

True. Proof of negligence in malpractice cases may be based on failure to obtain informed consent.

○ **What three things must be proven in order to prove malpractice based on lack of consent?**

1. That the provider failed to disclose all the material facts that a reasonable person would require to make an informed decision
2. That the patient's injury was caused by the provider's act, for which the patient granted uninformed permission
3. That a reasonable person would have withheld consent had the material facts been disclosed

○ **Since consent in CPR may be implied in cardiac arrest cases, when may problems arise?**

In emergency situations when documents on the victim's person or statements made by family members purport to represent the victim's intended refusal of CPR.

○ **What is the generally recognized practice in such situations?**

To initiate resuscitative efforts, with the understanding that CPR may be discontinued based on subsequent authentication of the patient's previously expressed wishes.

○ **May a hospital be liable for the organized services it provides and for the individual acts of its employees?**

Yes.

○ **What are the four legal requirements vis-à-vis CPR required of hospitals?**

To maintain sufficient personnel properly trained
To provide equipment
To implement an emergency alerting system within the hospital
To monitor performance

○ **Of what legal privilege does the above often deprive hospital personnel?**

The legal immunity available to out-of-hospital rescuers.

○   **What is the "captain-of-the-ship" doctrine?**

That a leader be held vicariously liable for the conduct of others in the group, depending on his or her level of control or right of control of the group members.

○   **How does this apply to CPR?**

Because customary practices include prompt designation of a leader from among the responders to a cardiac arrest.

○   **What is the modern legal trend in this regard?**

It is generally articulated with reference to surgical teams, recognizes the distinct areas of expertise contributed by each member, and tends to hold each to a standard of his or her class and ultimately his or her employer rather than shift liability to the team leader.

○   **Does traditional American law enforce the moral obligation to help others?**

No, it does not. Failure to act, however ignoble, may be above legal reproach.

○   **What kinds of personnel operate under an implied contract to act in an emergency?**

Emergency department healthcare providers, police, lifeguards, or EMTs.

○   **What sort of duty do special-status relationships, such as parent-child, captain-passenger, and employer-employee entail?**

A general legal duty to rescue if the effort can be made without endangering the rescuer.

○   **Do off-duty medical personnel have a duty to act in an emergency?**

While the moral obligation of providers to assist in emergencies is asserted in the professional code of ethics, no legal duty to act has been imposed simply because they are providers.

○   **Have any statutes requiring persons to offer emergency assistance been enacted?**

Yes, in Vermont and Minnesota. These may indicate a movement toward recognition of a general duty to rescue.

○   **Once you have initiated CPR, do you incur a legal liability to continue?**

Once steps are initiated and termination would place the victim in a worse position or compromise the likelihood of assistance from others, the potential rescuer incurs a legal duty to perform appropriately.

❍ **What is the purpose of Good Samaritan statutes?**

To protect health professionals and to encourage response by trained persons.

❍ **What is a common requirement of all Good Samaritan statutes?**

That the rescuer show "good faith" belief that the situation called for the immediate action undertaken.

❍ **Do most statutes grant legal immunity for incompetent rescue attempts?**

Yes, unless the actions would be considered reckless, offensive, and shocking to most people.

❍ **Do statutes cover events that take place during transport to a medical facility?**

Rescue settings vary by statute. In some states only actions at the site of the emergency are covered; other states include events during transport to a medical facility.

❍ **Do statutes extend immunity to persons responding to an emergency within a hospital?**

Some do, but only if they have no preexisting duty to offer assistance. In contrast, others deny protection to the same persons.

❍ **Why should first responders not fear litigation from making reasonable attempts at CPR?**

Because CPR attempts in emergencies are likely to be viewed as reasonable, even when provided by an inadequately trained rescuer, as long as there is a good-faith belief that the possible benefits of the attempt outweigh the risk from the rescuer's incompetence.

❍ **Should the first responder at the scene of a cardiac arrest assess resuscitability prior to initiating CPR?**

No, they are encouraged to initiate full CPR measures in virtually all instances.

❍ **Why is this?**

Because of the absence of accepted criteria for immediate determination of death, with few exceptions. A decision to terminate CPR based on nonresuscitability is equivalent to determining death and therefore must be made by a physician.

○   **What kind of information provided by bystanders should be ignored in making a decision as to whether to initiate CPR?**

Unreliable or unverifiable information about prior illness of the victim or about wishes previously expressed by the victim against CPR.

○   **How long must a nonphysician continue CPR?**

To the limits of their physical endurance or until the care of the victim is transferred to another qualified, responsible person.

○   **What attempts are states making to change this practice?**

An increasing number of states are exploring ways to authorize nonphysician emergency medical personnel to withhold or discontinue resuscitative efforts in the field based on criteria for poor survival or recognition of patients' requests not to resuscitate.

○   **Once started, how long must a physician continue to administer CPR?**

As necessary until the victim is transferred to the care of other properly trained personnel or until cardiac death (as defined by cardiovascular unresponsiveness to acceptable resuscitative techniques) is determined.

○   **What percent of deaths occur in hospitals?**

Approximately 80%.

○   **According to the National Conference Steering Committee, what is the purpose of CPR?**

The prevention of sudden, unexpected death.

○   **You are performing CPR on a terminal patient with end-stage renal disease. What right may you be violating?**

The individual's right to die with dignity.

○   **Where and by whom must contraindications to CPR be recorded in hospital?**

On the patient's chart by the attending physician.

○   **Must pre-hospital personnel honor hospital DNR orders?**

Many state laws still make it illegal for pre-hospital personnel to honor a hospital DNR order.

○   **Can a competent person refuse CPR?**

Consistent with the principle of self-determination, a competent patient's right to refuse CPR is virtually absolute.

○   **T/F: Court decisions have emphasized the same right of self-determination for incompetent patients with surrogate decision makers as for that granted for competent patients.**

True. Therefore, surrogate decision makers who are engaged in decisions about life sustaining treatment for incompetent patients are required to ascertain and represent the wishes expressed by the patient while the patient was still competent (e.g., "substituted judgment").

○   **When might it be impossible to ascertain the patient's prior wishes?**

If the patient was never competent, as in the case of minors.

○   **If the patient's prior wishes cannot be determined, how is resuscitation status determined?**

Physicians and surrogate decision makers may decide the resuscitation status based on their assessment of the patient's "best interests."

○   **How are conflicts between legitimate parental rights of family privacy and the state's interest in protecting the welfare of children decided?**

On whether life-sustaining treatment serves the best interest of an individual child.

○   **What two important elements should hospital policies governing orders not to resuscitate contain?**

1. Requirements that do-not-resuscitate orders be written on the order sheet, accompanied by progress notes that explain the rationale for the decision and identify the participants in the decision-making process
2. Guidelines for prior judicial review in specifically enumerated circumstances

○   **What are "partial code" orders?**

Orders that limit the extent of resuscitation to be offered a patient.

○   **What is the purpose of establishing ethics committees at hospitals?**

To provide more systematic and disciplined approaches to medical decision making.

○   **What are the four main functions of the ethics committee?**

Education
Consultation
Development of hospital policies and guidelines

Case reviews

○ **On what does the paramedic's scope of practice rely?**

Standing order protocols and offline medical direction (indirect medical control).

○ **May an EMT disregard or countermand an order given by a physician?**

Not as a rule. However, most EMS systems have specific policies dealing with this issue. The procedure used varies widely from system to system.

○ **What recent developments have challenged traditional legal, cultural and religious concepts of death?**

Technology that may maintain cardiorespiratory function in patients with minimal or no brain function and no possibility of recovery.

○ **What has become well established in the United States as a legal standard of death?**

That death of the whole brain has occurred.

○ **What one of two conditions must be met to conform to the Model Uniform Determination of Death Act?**

Irreversible cessation of circulation and respiratory function or
Irreversible cessation of all functions of the entire brain including the brain stem

○ **What is the controversial "conscience clause" enacted in New Jersey?**

In situations in which the physician is aware that the patient's or family's religious convictions would be violated by a declaration of brain death, only cardiorespiratory death criteria may be applied.

○ **T/F: Criteria developed for brain death in adults and children are the same.**

False. Specific criteria for brain death developed for adults have not been validated for children.

○ **Diagnosis of death based on neurological criteria should be approached with particular caution in certain circumstances, such as . . .**

Hypothermia
Use of neuromuscular blocking agents or barbiturates
Unknown cause of brain insult

○ **T/F: Cardiopulmonary support systems may be withdrawn from brain-dead patients without judicial review or fear of legal repercussions.**

True.

○   **Does the discontinuance of cardiorespiratory support systems for brain-dead patients affect an assailant's charges or defense in homicide or child abuse cases?**

No. Courts have consistently rejected such arguments and have authorized the discontinuation of life-support.

○   **If a conflict arises between the rights of a mother and her fetus in regard to maternal resuscitation, who wins?**

These are rare cases, and there is insufficient case law to offer a definitive answer.

○   **In regard to CPR, what does the Patient Self-determination act passed by Congress in 1990 require?**

That hospitals and other health care facilities and agencies that participate in Medicare and Medicaid establish written policies and procedures to inform all adult patients of their right to prescribe binding limits to CPR and life-sustaining measures in the event of future decisional incapacity.

○   **What did the 1991 revision of this Act require?**

That hospitals and healthcare agencies establish written policies and procedures to inform all adult patients of their rights to make decisions concerning medical care, including the right to accept or refuse medical or surgical treatment and the right to formulate an advanced directive.

○   **What is the largest single source of malpractice suits against pediatricians?**

Birth-related problems.

○   **What are "required request" laws in regard to organ donations?**

Laws that require documentation that families of potential donors are offered the option of organ donation and that the local organ procurement organization is notified of potential donors.

○   **What is the controversial proposal for "presumed consent"?**

This would permit the body of every deceased person to be used as a potential organ donor unless that person had declared an objection to being a donor before death, or the next of kin declares such an objection immediately upon notification of death.

○   **Have such decrees been adopted?**

Yes, in several countries, but not in the United States.

○   **Is it ethical to practice intubation skills on newly deceased infants and children?**

This practice, although controversial, is brief and beneficial to others and is an effective teaching technique. However, the sensibilities of family and staff should be respected and consent obtained.

BIBLIOGRAPHY

Chameides, Leon and Mary Fran Hazinski, eds. *Pediatric Advanced Life Support.* Dallas: American Heart Association, 2002.

Guidelines 2000 for Cardiopulmonary Resuscitation and Emergency Cardiac Care: An International Consensus on Science. *Circulation* 2000; 102:8 (suppl I): 1-I-370.

Hazinski, Mary Fran, et al., eds. *2000 Handbook of Emergency Cardiovascular Care for Healthcare Providers.* Dallas: American Heart Association, 2000.

"Part 10: Pediatric Advanced Life Support," *Circulation* 2000; 102 (suppl. I): I-291—I234.

NOTES

NOTES

NOTES

NOTES

NOTES